Releasing Emotional Patterns
with
Essential Oils

Published by: VisionWare Press
                 P.O. Box 8112
                 Rancho Santa Fe, CA 92067

The oils listed are the trademarks of Young Living Essential Oils. For further information, contact your Young Living Distributor.

First Printing, July 1998
Revised Edition, August 1999
Third Edition, October 2000
Fourth Edition, January 2002
Fifth Edition, January 2004
Sixth Edition, March 2005
Seventh Edition, January 2007
Eighth Edition, August 2008
Ninth Edition, January 2011
Tenth Edition, May 2012
Eleventh Edition, January 2014
Twelfth Edition, January 2015
Thirteenth Edition, January 2017

Printed in the United States of America.

Copyright © 1998 by Carolyn L. Mein, D.C.

ISBN 978-1-5426908-1-2

Art work by Richard Alan.

DEDICATION

I dedicate this book to those who are seeking
additional ways to use essential oils for emotional healing.

TABLE OF CONTENTS

PREFACE

Many years ago I heard that the quickest way to self-realization and ultimately spiritual oneness was through service, especially healing. As I began my chiropractic career, I was continually shown the validity of this statement in increased awareness for myself, as well as my patients' personal awareness. Illness has a way of showing us what is real, forcing us to honor ourselves and take personal responsibility for our thoughts and actions. Likewise, healing, whether it be through our own experience or that of another, brings valuable insights and awareness.

The illness that characteristically forces us to look at all aspects of our being is cancer. The prevention and various cures of cancer have been one of my interests, since my father died of cancer the year I graduated from chiropractic college; he was only 45 years of age. It was my interest in the early detection and treatment of cancer that lead me to meet Dr. D. Gary Young when he had his clinics in Chula Vista, California and Mexico. I was impressed by his research, dedication, and sincerity. It was only natural for him to eventually focus on prevention and make the healing properties of essential oils, and how to use them, available to the general public.

Knowing that if there was a question, there had to be an answer, I set out to discover the most effective ways of healing and maintaining health. This led me into acupuncture, nutrition, Applied Kinesiology, numerous other forms of healing, and the development of Transpersonal Physiology. In an attempt to understand the different dietary needs of my patients, I discovered that the body is regulated or controlled by a dominant gland, organ or system. This is what determines and explains why there are varying weight gain patterns, physical characteristics and obvious differences in people's dietary needs. There are actually 25 distinct body types. Not only do they have different dietary requirements, they have different psychological profiles which are expressed in their characteristic traits and motivations. The 25 Body Type System is really a bridge between our ultimate goal of unconditional love and spiritual oneness, and our day-to-day reality. Since our bodies contain our history and provide constant feedback, learning to listen to them provides a natural guide. Noticing your body's response to your diet and being aware of its moods is an ideal place to start. Your psychological profile allows you to understand what motivates you, describes your unique gifts, and enhances self-esteem.

While people have different motivations for their behavior and different dominant traits, they all have access to all the emotions. It was through Transpersonal Physiology that I was able to identify a vibrational frequency for physical conditions and emotional patterns. A disruption in the body can be corrected by balancing energy using acupuncture points. This was the basis of clearing the physical aspect of emotional patterns. The use of essential oils adds another dimension by providing access to the limbic system of the brain. One of my patients, Linda Lull, found she could use the organ alarm points, with the associated emotions and oils, to enhance her balance and harmony for the day. As a result of her experience and sharing it with others, including Dr. Terry Friedmann, this portion of my research is available for your information and use. It is intended to provide guidelines for a more specific use of the essential oils with particular emphasis on their emotional applications.

Carolyn L. Mein, D.C.

ACKNOWLEDGEMENTS

I would like to acknowledge all those who have contributed to the additions for this new edition of *Releasing Emotional Patterns with Essential Oils*. To my students, colleagues, and patients for their questions and insights.

To all of you who have used the first and revised editions of this book and for your willing participation and feedback. To Kalee Gracse for identifying related control issues. To Fawn Christianson for identifying additional emotions. To Sonoma Selena for her list of additional words relating to underlying emotions. To Kathy Farmer for her additions and clearing procedure. To Susan Ulfelder for her research and input on her alternative clearing method. To Connie and Alan Higley for their Ear Chart. To Dr. Gary Young, N.D. for the formulation of the essential oil blends, providing consistent therapeutic quality oils, his writing technique for clearing, and ongoing support.

To Jeannie Keller for typing and formatting, to Craig Ridgley for his computer expertise, to Francis Bischetti for his continuous updating and support, and Nadine Mein for proofing.

Emotional Clearing

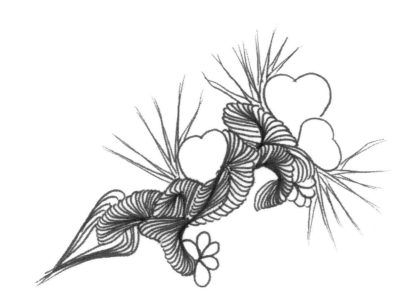

RELEASING EMOTIONAL PATTERNS
WITH ESSENTIAL OILS

Do you find yourself at the mercy of your emotions?

Is shifting out of a negative emotional state difficult?

Do you get pulled into the emotional vortex of those around you?

Do you find yourself repeatedly responding in the same negative way to some situations regardless of your best intentions to do otherwise?

Do your negative emotions seem to be beyond your control?

Emotions are like ocean waves–they ebb and flow. They are powerful and provide momentum initiating action. Most of us are aware of the negative side of an emotion, but rarely do we know the positive or other side, let alone how to access it. For example, we have all experienced anger, but what is the opposite or positive emotion, and how do we get there, especially when we are embroiled in anger. The expression of the negative side of an emotion is usually painful; consequently, we develop defenses to protect ourselves. One of the most common defenses is to ignore, repress or stuff our negative emotions. What happens when we stuff negative emotions? They are held in the body and eventually produce physical or emotional pain.

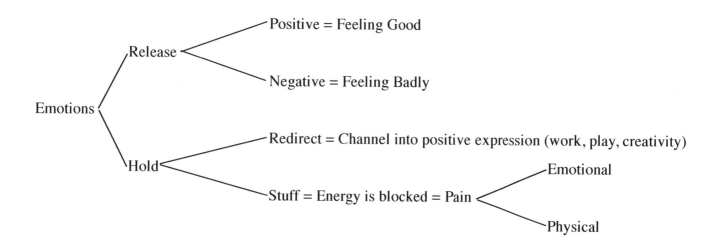

Emotions have a negative and positive polarity. We need to be able to access both polarities of all our emotions to be fully alive. Avoiding situations that could cause emotional pain limits our life experiences.

Since holding on to negative emotions has adverse effects on the body, what happens when these emotions are released? While you may feel better initially, if the emotional expression is negative, there are usually repercussions.

The alternative to a negative response is to express the positive side of the emotion. That sounds like a viable option, so let's take a common emotion like anger. We all know how it feels to get angry and what it is like to be the recipient of someone else's anger. Now that we have decided to express the positive or other side, what is it? Joy, happiness, love, peace? While these are all positive emotions, is any one of them the opposite of anger?

To find a positive expression for the energy known as anger, we need to understand what it is and what causes it. Let's say you are pursuing your goal. You are picking up momentum and everything is moving along just fine when you suddenly hit a roadblock. Your options are to go over it, under it, around it or through it. If you are not sure of which direction to go, you will sit there trying to decide as the energy continues to build. When the pressure reaches a sufficient level, something has to give way. The negative expression of this energy is anger.

Anger doesn't always have to have a negative effect. It could provide the impetus to change an unhealthy situation or bring a problem into conscious awareness so a solution can be found. Regardless, anger is an explosion of energy that gets attention. What is a positive expression of an explosion of energy? Laughter. Now, what would you rather experience, anger or laughter?

Wait a minute, what happens if you have a lot of negative energy around a positive emotion? Perhaps you were told your laughter was inappropriate or were laughed at as a child. If this were the case, it would be hard for you to spontaneously laugh. Accessing your laughter requires releasing the blocked emotions around laughter as well as around anger.

When you are able to feel both sides of the emotion, you are free to fully experience the feeling. You now have a choice of holding or releasing the emotion. Releasing the emotion positively creates good feelings for yourself and those around you. Holding the positive emotion allows you to use the energy for a positive or creative expression through work or play.

Aspects of Clearing Emotional Patterns
Changing an emotional pattern takes more than just feeling both sides of the emotion. It takes recognizing and understanding the pattern that triggers the emotion, which is the mental aspect. It takes getting the message or learning the lesson by increasing awareness, which is the spiritual aspect. Changing the automatic conditioned response requires accessing the cellular memory that is stored in the physical body.

While the decision to change a pattern is the first step, it alone is not enough to shift a well-ingrained response. The pattern needs to be understood and identified so it can be recognized. Once you are able to recognize an emotional pattern, like anger, you can decide whether you want to feel anger or laughter. Let's say you would like to feel laughter, but you can't seem to get past the anger. Knowing that anger comes from your direction being blocked, you need to change your perspective to see the situation from a different point of view, enabling you to determine your way out or the best direction to take. This higher perspective is the spiritual component that provides the "way out" and allows you to get the message or

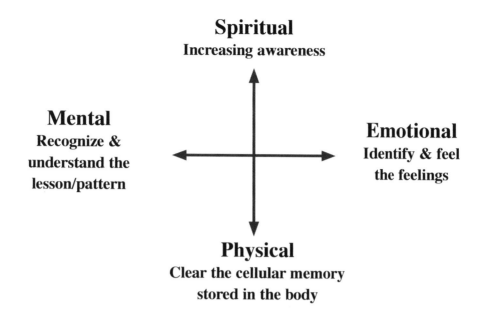

Spiritual
Increasing awareness

Mental
**Recognize &
understand the
lesson/pattern**

Emotional
**Identify & feel
the feelings**

Physical
**Clear the cellular memory
stored in the body**

Effectively clearing emotional patterns requires accessing all four areas.

lesson by increasing your awareness. The "way out" of anger is to shift perspective. "My direction is clear" facilitates the shift. Automatic responses have a physical component, meaning the emotion is stored in the cells of the body. We know from traditional acupuncture that anger is stored in the liver. The liver, as well as the other glands and organs, can be accessed through points on the body known as alarm points.

Essential Oils To Release Or Change Emotional Patterns

Have you ever noticed how smells, like bread baking, can send you back to a childhood memory and all the feelings associated with your favorite grandmother? Smell accesses the limbic system of the brain which is the seat of our emotions[1]. Ancient Egyptians used essential oils to clear specific emotions and recorded them on the walls of certain temple healing chambers.

Sesquiterpenes, found in high levels in essential oils such as Frankincense and Sandalwood, help to increase the oxygen in the limbic system of the brain which in turn "unlocks" the DNA and allows emotional baggage to be released from cellular memory. Emotions have been found to be encoded within the DNA of the cells and passed on from generation to generation. Emotional behavior patterns have even been found to be "locked" within families. Transplant recipients report strange memories and desires which further substantiates that emotions are stored in the body and encoded in the DNA of the cells[2]. More recently, studies at New York University proved the amygdala gland (the gland in the limbic system of the brain that stores and releases trauma in the body) does not respond to sound or sight or touch, but ONLY releases emotional trauma through the sense of smell.[3]

---

[1] *Molecules of Emotion*, Candace B. Peri, Ph.D

[2] *The Heart Code*, Paul P. Pearsall

[3] *Unlocking Emotions with Essential Oils*, Kathy Farmer

Emotions themselves are stored in the body in its organs, glands, and systems. Feelings are taken in through the chakras, or energy centers along the midline of the body, and then fed into the meridian system, which consists of energy channels that run over and through the body. Since each organ has a vibrational frequency, as do emotions, the emotions will settle in an area with a corresponding frequency. Disease occurs when the body's vibrational frequency drops below a certain point. Essential oils can raise the body's frequency, and therapeutic grade (medicinal quality) oils are able to do this because they vibrate at a high frequency and transfer that frequency to the body.

Essential oils have been used throughout the ages for healing, and the Bible contains 188 references to them. For example, *Frankincense, Myrrh, Rosemary, Hyssop*, and *Spikenard* were oils used for anointing and healing the sick in Biblical times. One of the oldest healing modalities known, acupuncture, uses the emotions associated with, and stored in, the major organs to diagnose disease.

Cause of Emotional Patterns

An emotional pattern is a fear-based survival response. The purpose of the ego is to protect us from harm. The ego is like a big computer; it collects all the data from our life's experiences, takes everything that is said literally and stores it. The ego's protective responses are based on past experiences, so future responses will be the same unless the program is changed. As we mature and grow we need to update the ego's program to experience our full potential.

For example, when you were a small child, you were told not to go into the street. When you were older and able to be responsible for yourself, you were taught to look both ways and to cross the street when it was safe. If you stayed with the initial program of "The street is dangerous, stay out of it," you would be afraid to cross the street and never experience the world beyond the block where you lived.

As children, we make survival decisions based on our abilities. If you grew up with parents that would punish you every time you said something they didn't like, you would quickly learn to keep your parents happy by not expressing your feelings whenever you thought it would upset them. This would initiate a survival pattern of not speaking your truth when the people around you could disapprove.

To be safe you had to control your emotions. Since it wasn't safe to spontaneously express your feelings, you had to suppress and internalize them or find another outlet. As children, we have limited resources, especially when our role models have poor ways of handling their negative emotions. As a result, most of us know the negative expression of an emotion but few of us know the positive side, let alone how to access it.

Pain is usually what causes us to seek better ways of handling situations. Pain is usually induced through trauma either physical or emotional. The trauma then initiates an emotional pattern, which causes the following to occur.

1. The emotional energy that gets generated during the trauma enters the body and, if it is not released, gets stored in an organ or gland with the same vibrational energy. For example, anger is stored in the liver.

2. The memory of the trauma gets stored in the limbic system of the brain, which is the seat of the emotions.

3. Our minds create a belief and attach it to the emotional memory stored in the limbic system of the brain.

4. The emotional response to the trauma gets stored in the cellular memory throughout the body and becomes automatic.

Identifying Emotional Patterns

The easiest way to identify emotional patterns is through your feelings. While a trauma, either real or perceived, will set up the initial pattern, similar situations trigger the pattern, providing an opportunity to either perpetuate or heal it.

Anything that bothers you carries an emotional charge. As your awareness grows, you have more resources to handle a situation differently, learning from your past experiences. If you choose to ignore and suppress the feelings, the problem tends to magnify each time it presents itself.

The essence of our life experience is to have experiences so we can learn, grow and master. The experiences we learn most from are the ones that get our attention. For most of us, it takes pain to cause us to look at a situation. However, all too often emotional trauma produces more pain than we can deal with, so we block it off from our conscious awareness. Since we are supposed to get wiser as we get older, learning from life's experiences, the unhealed emotional trauma eventually resurfaces. Why? Because there is something we need to learn. What is the basic lesson? To come from love, rather than fear. All emotions stem from either love or fear. Fear ultimately comes from a disconnection with one's spiritual source.

Consequently, all religions and spiritual paths point to a Supreme Spiritual Being as the source of all that is. The goal is spiritual connection which is reflected in the way we live our lives. Essentially, being spiritually aligned allows one to come from love and express the positive qualities of life.

The body holds emotional patterns regardless of conscious awareness. Since the body never lies and holds blocked energy, it is a good indicator of unresolved emotional issues. Often times, the first indication of a problem is pain–physical, emotional or both. Many physical problems have an emotional component, especially when they are chronic. Some emotions are so strong and evident that they are easy to recognize. When this is the case, you can approach the emotion by going to the specific emotion found in the Emotional Reference section and begin directly releasing it.

Sometimes we bury our emotions and they are stored in the body until sufficient pressure builds, producing pain or disease in the area[4]. To identify the emotion associated with a particular area of pain, locate the pain on the body charts and refer to the Body Reference for the associated emotion.

---

[4] *Feelings Buried Alive Never Die*, Carol Truman

Once the emotion has been identified, its other side understood, and the lesson or the way out known, it needs to be released from cellular memory. Caroline Myss, Ph.D.[5] states that 70% of the body's cells need to shift before a new direction becomes a reality. This explains why it takes more than conscious awareness for a pattern to shift. While understanding a problem is important, the body or cellular memory needs to get the message as well, hence the need for repetition of the clearing procedure.

Identifying Core Issues

When identifying an emotional pattern, the most effective way of changing the pattern is to be as specific as possible in getting to the core issue. If you are using muscle testing, which is a way of connecting with your subconscious and is described in the last chapter, as a way of pinpointing the issue, you will find related areas that are close. Your indication of an emotion that is close, but not the main issue, is that the muscle will test "spongy" rather than solidly strong or weak. Certain emotions like bitterness and hate relate to deeper issues and are referenced as *see past* or *see anger*. Continuing to explore for the deeper emotion allows you to locate the core issue. Working with this issue allows you to maximize your efficiency. However, there are related emotions to each core issue. Working with the surrounding emotions allows you to reduce the emotional intensity.

Dealing With Related Emotions

When dealing with a core issue, one that requires applying the essential oil and doing the emotional repatterning 18 times a day for seven weeks, it is common to have associated emotions surface in the process. If desired, you may add related emotions using different oils before you have completed the seven weeks, or you may work with these related emotions using the same oil. For example, you may start with *Lavender* to repattern "fear of criticism" and add "fear of abandonment" to the procedure before you are finished with the first emotion.

During the clearing process you may experience emotions surfacing quickly or intensely. If using the oil brings up more emotions than you feel you can handle, take a break and process the emotions in a time frame that is comfortable. When you are ready to continue, pick up where you left off. Overwhelming emotions generally indicate underlying emotions that also need to be cleared. Working with them along with the core issues often reduces the overwhelming emotions. As memories and emotions surface, it is often helpful to write, go for a walk, meditate, talk to a close friend, or exercise. More information on writing techniques is found in the Clearing Enhancements section.

---

[5] *Why People Don't Heal And How They Can*, Caroline Myss. Ph.D

CLEARING EMOTIONAL PATTERNS

Emotional patterns are held in cellular memory and affect us physically, mentally and emotionally. Changing behavior patterns requires:

1. **Understanding the emotional pattern.** This involves seeing how the same emotion presents itself in different situations and how it affects your life. It allows you to see why you are experiencing the problems in your life. Once the pattern is understood or the issue is defined, the message or a better way of handling the situation appears.

2. **Recognize the problem** before you find yourself in the middle of it. By understanding the cause of the problem, situations can be dealt with in a better way. In essence, the lesson has been learned.

3. **Being willing and ready to change.** Until the ramifications or effects of a behavior are understood or experienced, there is no need, requirement, or motivation to change. This fact is why situations get worse or deteriorate to an unbearable level before a person is able to see the pattern and his/her role in it. Change requires a shifting of direction, which takes effort and focused energy.

4. **Changing the emotional energy pattern.** An automatic behavior or response is a fixed energy pattern. To effectively make a change, the energy needs to be cleared out of all parts of the body: physical, mental and emotional. Learning the lesson affects the spiritual body; understanding the pattern addresses the mental body; the associated alarm points acess the physical body; and feelings relate to the emotional body.

Clearing Patterns

Clearing a deep pattern requires bringing the lesson to conscious awareness and fully understanding it, essentially learning the lesson. Clearing the emotional pattern from the body requires feeling the emotion and releasing it from the body's cellular memory. Emotions stored in the glands and organs can be accessed through the acupuncture alarm points, and the limbic system accessed through smell. Essential oils hold vibrational frequencies that can shift patterns. Using them on the acupuncture alarm points sends the frequency directly to the specific organ and smelling the oil releases the pattern from the limbic system of the brain, thus providing direct access to the body's cellular memory.

Releasing emotional patterns requires:

1) identifying the pattern that is linked to the emotion,

2) understanding the pattern—the opposite side of the emotion,

3) learning the lesson by discovering the way out of the situation,

4) clearing and reprogramming the pattern in the body's cellular memory—changing DNA, and

5) releasing the pattern from the memory held in the limbic system of the brain.

What to Expect

Clearing emotional patterns with essential oils is very gentle.

Changes are often subtle because the body is able to release the programming in the same way it came in, one step at a time. This is the reason for the repetition. The length of time is immaterial. You can move at your own pace, whether you take 7 weeks or 7 months to clear a core issue is up to you. Learning how to shift from the negative to the positive emotion makes the changes permanent.

You will find yourself responding to situations rather than reacting. There is often a sense of inner peace, deep relaxation, or an opening, allowing your body to breathe. You will notice more flexibility which is evidenced by the way you handle situations.

Emotions, memories and being aware surface when you are able to handle them. The clearing process starts with a painful emotion like rejection, and moves you into a positive state. While the statement, "I accept all that I am," can bring up all the "yes, but" responses of the internal dialogue committee, the end result is a state of acceptance. As you continue the repetition process you eventually erase the old cellular response pattern and replace it with the new one of acceptance.

Our challenge is to express love regardless of what life presents. The game is survival with our greatest fears as the stage. Fear is the cause of emotional patterns, also known as psychological issues, which reflect the lessons each of us has to learn. While we all have all the emotional patterns, some of them are more of a challenge than others. Some patterns are universal, while others are more common for certain people than others. There is a common denominator among groups of people and it is reflected in their body shape. Hence the stereo-type of fat people being jolly and skinny people being more serious. Body shape is determined by the gland, organ or system of the body that is the most dominant. This dominant gland controls not only body shape, but basic personality traits.

Emotional patterns are stored in the body with major life challenges correlating with each person's dominant gland that determines his/her body type. How to determine body type and the main issues associated with each type are found in Points of Connection. The following typical experiences show the effect clearing emotional patterns has on one's life.

Typical Experiences

Anger

Lane is a twenty-six year old man whose dominant gland and body type is Thymus. The core issues or major challenges of the Thymus Body Type are judgement and control, with anger being the dominant emotional response. He began using the essential oil blend of *Purification* on the liver alarm points and the emotional points at the frontal eminences seven times a day along with feeling the emotions of anger, then laughter, and making the statement, "My direction is clear."

In less than a week, he experienced his favorite guitar being knocked over and the case chipped while at band practice. His normal response to situations like this would be intense anger that permeated everyone in his environment and continued for at least a week before any solution could begin to surface.

This time he walked into the house and told his mother he was angry because his guitar had been chipped. Within the hour he was out in the garage, had found some black paint, and repaired the chipped spot to where it was almost undetectable. This incident has been followed by similar situations where he has been able to quickly move out of an anger response, and even bypass the anger, to reach a viable solution that works for everyone.

Once he finished using the *Purification* oil for three weeks, the next emotion, frustration which is stored in the common bile duct, surfaced. The "other side" of frustration is accomplishment. The "way out" is, "I move beyond my limitations." Having finished using *Lemon* oil seven times a day for three weeks, he was then ready to deal with the core issue for the Thymus Body Type, fear of failure. The "other side" of fear of failure is unfoldment and the "way out" is, "I accept growth". The alarm point is the thymus and the essential oil is *Peppermint*.

Clearing the emotional patterns with the "way out" and essential oils has allowed Lane to transform core issues and change emotional responses he had been dealing with his entire life. He has been able to easily integrate the new patterns into his being, making his life easier and happier as a result.

Relationships

Molly is a forty-year old woman who has done a lot of personal growth work, including psychotherapy, for years. While she thoroughly understood the dynamics of her relationships, she was unable to break the emotional patterns that bound her. She started using *Lavender* to clear her deep-seated abandonment issues along with the statement, "I learn from all of life's experiences."

Shortly thereafter, she found herself in a situation with her boyfriend where she felt compelled to express her feelings rather than continue to keep them bottled up inside herself. The next morning, she felt fabulous and self-empowered. Her boyfriend wanted to end the relationship. For the first time in her life, she was able to say and mean, "If that's what you really want and need for yourself, I'll respect your decision." In spite of the fact that she missed him and knew it was the right decision, this was the first time she was able to go through a breakup without engaging her abandonment issues and begging for her lover to come back. She attributed it all to clearing her emotional pattern of abandonment.

Chronic Illness

The body is a wonderful indicator of what is going on in a person's life. It reflects physically what is occurring emotionally, in spite of what the mind does to rationalize or ignore reality. Tatiana's body responded by forming visible tumors. The initial one appeared in 1989 on the bottom of her foot. She sought conventional medical help and had the tumor and a portion of her foot removed. Being a professional dancer, she realized this was a wake-up call that resulted in her leaving a bad marriage.

In 1996, a number of years later when she noticed a couple of tumors on her leg, she realized she needed to get to the cause of the problem rather than just treat the symptoms. This was the beginning of her journey into personal growth and psychotherapy. When the tumors appeared the third time, in 1999, Tatiana identified a common thread. Each time the tumors appeared Tatiana was in a relationship with a man where she had given up her identity. In the past she had left each relationship knowing that in spite of the emotional pain, it was what she had to do to survive.

This time Tatiana had another tool, the knowledge of how to use essential oils to release deep emotional patterns. She recognized a number of related emotional patterns and used the corresponding essential oils and clearing procedure. Tatiana was sporadic with her use of some of the oils with little noticeable difference except for two: *Release* for fear of love not being unconditional and *Lavender* for her fear of abandonment. When she used *Lavender*, Tatiana was amazed to feel her abandonment pain dissipate. This was the first time she was able to leave a relationship and feel whole. She got through the entire breakup without crying and going back on what she knew was right for her. Daniel, the man she was in a relationship with, initiated the break-up because Tatiana was giving too much of her energy to him and he could see that it was impacting her healing. She was drawing him in to complete herself and coming up against her fear of commitment. As soon as Tatiana got home, she began applying *Release* and *Lavender* and saying the Forgiveness Prayer every time she thought about Daniel. She did the prayer and the oils approximately every hour and was amazed at how well she slept that night as well as how easily she got through the next three days.

The Forgiviness Prayer Tatiana used is by Dr. Roberta Herzog. It is reprinted by permission. See resources for additional information.

The Law of Forgiveness
The Law of Forgiveness comes from "The Lord's Prayer" wherein it is said, "...and forgive us our trespasses as we forgive those who trespass against us..." This is a Universal Law... that when you forgive and ask for forgiveness in return, the Karma of the situation begins to be neutralized.

Here is what you can do to help yourself: Every morning and every evening for *At Least* 10 Days to 2 weeks, when you rise in the morning and before retiring at night, sit and be still. Close your eyes. Picture the soul that you wish to forgive smiling and happy. Then say the following, out loud, to this soul:

"_____, I forgive you for *Everything* you've ever said or done to me in thought, word or deed that has caused me pain in this or any other lifetime. You are free and I am free! And _____, I ask that you forgive *Me* for *Anything* that I have ever said or done to you in thought, word or deed in this or any other lifetime that has caused you pain. You are free and I am free! Thank you, God, for this opportunity to forgive _____ and to forgive myself."

You will "Know" when to cease saying this on a daily basis when you have a *True Release* sometime after 10 days to 2 weeks. That release may be crying, laughter, a feeling of well-being...anything. You will also find that *You Have Entirely Changed Your Attitude Towards This Soul* and that this soul's *Attitude Will Change Towards You, Too!* You will now begin to really see what the problem is and begin to *Work With That Karma* and neutralize it, freeing yourself from pain, becoming happier, healthier and more peaceful in mind, body and spirit.

Tatiana realized she had been trying to complete herself with someone else. Her belief was, "If I give you what you want, you will love me. If I complete you by providing fulfilling sex, you will complete me and take care of me." Tatiana realized she didn't need a sexual relationship to be complete. She needed to take responsibility for herself so she added *Birch*. Once she was able to change her focus from being half a person into being a whole person, she changed her experience with Daniel. They continued to see each other socially and Tatiana noticed they were becoming two complete energies within themselves that came together to create a third energy.

Being a Stomach Body Type, *Peace and Calming* was extremely valuable for her fear of losing control. Abandonment during an illness or crisis is a fear Tatiana has carried as long as she can remember. Once she recognized the profound effect the *Lavender* had on her abandonment issue, Tatiana was able to address other issues as well and allow them to clear just as gently. Tatiana now has a profound sense of inner knowing that she has learned the lesson of keeping the commitment to take care of herself and has changed the cellular pattern that led to her body's tumor formation.

Abundance

Pete, a self-employed contractor, Adrenal Body Type, age forty-five, wanted to work on abundance. Being self-employed, he was responsible for procuring all the jobs for himself and his crew. We began by testing for abundance which did not show up; then lack which also tested negative. Looking for the underlying emotion, we found failure. Fear of failure is stored in the thymus gland. The other side of failure is unfoldment, and the way to get to unfoldment is "I accept growth". The quickest way for Pete to change this pattern was to apply *Peppermint* oil, feel the feelings, and say the statement, "I accept growth" 7 times per day for 7 weeks.

After 3 weeks, Pete had secured two large jobs that would keep him and his crew busy until the end of the year, in addition to his regular jobs. He realized that bringing in more business would require hiring more crew, so he decided to discontinue the *Peppermint* for a while. He decided he would resume the *Peppermint* when he was ready to accept growth in other areas of his life.

Ready for Change

Tanya realized she was in a verbally abusive relationship with her husband's teenage daughter, Suzie. Her husband's guilt over the divorce of Suzie's mother prevented him from disciplining her. The husband would not support or rescue Tanya from Suzie's anger and verbal abuse.

Tanya had "had it" with the dysfunction in her life and realized that the only way real healing could occur was for her to change her limiting patterns. She began by selecting two oils, *Purification* for anger and *SARA* for abuse, both connected with core issues to use 18 times a day for 7 weeks, along with a third oil, *Release*, to use 10 times a day for 7 weeks for loss of identity and fear of success. Being committed, her focus was on remembering to apply the oils. This was a full time job and a bit challenging when she wore a one piece leotard or pantyhose with a full length dress, especially since one of the issues was anger (liver alarm point) and another loss of identity (uterus alarm point).

The first week she only applied the oils 10 times a day rather than 18. As Tanya became aware of how she had not been valuing herself, she was able to increase the number to 18. Repeating the negative/old pattern followed by the positive/new state and the affirmation/statement brought her daily thought patterns into conscious awareness. She became aware of the direction she needed to go to get to where she wanted to be and what she had been doing to stay stuck. The old pattern of doing a little of everything without focus was associated with a fear of completion. This and other related patterns surfaced in a gentle way, at a pace she was able to handle. Dedicated to reaching a new plateau, she was aware of how good it felt to really care about herself as she continued the 7 weeks. Her newfound clarity and awareness allowed her to finally embark on a career.

Tanya had been raised to be selfless, of endless service and had become a doormat in the process. Using the oils, she immediately noticed she was able to calmly and efficiently handle situations where before she would react emotionally, especially with two teenagers in the house. Tanya was able to respond rationally, rather than react emotionally to stress, enabling her to maintain her peaceful place so she could step out of an argument rather than get caught up in it. With her body type being Lung, which is extremely sensitive to emotions, this was a major accomplishment. She gained greater clarity, self awareness, and strength. By lovingly and firmly expressing herself, her family gained a better understanding of how she really felt and developed a greater respect for her. Emotional by nature, clearing the negativity around core issues allowed her to get in touch with her true feelings and as a result, be true to herself.

Following her 7 week intensive, Tanya's purpose continues to become clearer and more defined as life presents her with opportunities to experience and express her gifts and talents. She is more and more aware of what she really wants to do. For the first time in her life she is finding her inner strength, her core, and integrating all aspects of herself. She has come to realize how who she is and how she r sponds to situations affects her family and every other person she contacts. While she is fully aware of the emotional state of those around her, she no longer has to emotionally reflect their emotions. For the first time in her life, she is set free.

Helping a Mate

Elaine and Bob have a very good, loving relationship. Even though they are exceptionally supportive of each other, there are times when Elaine feels that Bob doesn't listen to her. She has asked him repeatedly to please open her bathroom door when he gets up because she doesn't want to wake him with the noise of her hair dryer and the bathroom gets hot, but she can't hear him over the noise of the dryer. Even though he repeatedly promises to do better, he can't seem to remember to open the door. Another problem is the cat is getting old and finicky about her food. Elaine has repeatedly asked Bob not to give the cat so much food because she won't eat leftovers. Bob keeps giving her too much food and when reminded, feels Elaine is nagging him. When Elaine needs someone just to listen and shares her feelings of frustration, Bob gets upset, even angry at times, leaving Elaine feeling she can't share her feelings with him. Repeated discussion of the behavior pattern did nothing to change it, only brought up more frustration or aggravated the problem.

In talking to Elaine, I asked her what she felt the underlying issue was for Bob. She related it to his feeling helpless, like when his mother or his buddies in Vietnam were dying. The underlying emotion for feeling helpless is *overwhelmed*. The other side of *overwhelmed* is *vision* and the way to get there is with the statement, "I focus my energy." The oil is *Envision* and the alarm point is the vision point near the eyes.

Elaine shared her discovery with Bob and gave him the *Envision* oil. Elaine noticed that Bob put the statement with the emotions on his mirror. By the second morning, Elaine came to Bob and said, "It's working." The cat had the right amount of food, her door was open and their communication more free and open. Bob hadn't noticed the change yet, but did by the fifth day. Needless to say, Bob continued to use the oil and clear the pattern.

CLEARING EMOTIONAL PATTERNS

An emotional pattern may be identified from the emotion itself or from the area of the body where there is pain or discomfort. The Emotional Reference lists the emotions (both polarities), body alarm points, and the essential oils used to clear the patterns. Refer to the Charts section for the locations of the body alarm points.

The majority of the words listed under emotions are of the negative polarity. The ones that are positive relate to the fear of—such as the fear of love, not being loved, or not being lovable.

To clear an emotional pattern, begin by:

1) Identifying the feeling or emotion. This brings it into conscious awareness.

2) Once it has been identified, the emotion and the thought pattern that created it needs to be understood.

3) Next look at the "other side" or positive emotion, which is the gift or positive expression of the emotion.

4) The "way out" is a statement or affirmation that provides a way to shift the energy from the negative to positive. It focuses on the essence of the lesson so it can be easily seen and understood. Once the "way out" of a negative feeling is known, it is easy to shift out of an undesirable emotional state. When the negative emotion has lost its hold, and the lesson has been learned, then the related life situation is free to shift. If the negative emotion or situation reappears, the tools are in place to quickly shift one's attention and focus. This allows a position of choice and personal empowerment.

Clearing deep-seated emotional patterns requires releasing held emotional patterns and replacing them with the desired response. Changing a pattern is like filling in a groove–the deeper the groove, the more often you need to connect with the other side of the emotion. The "way out" provides the bridge that allows you to shift from the negative to the positive side of the emotion. The deeper the emotional pattern, the more often you need to link both sides of the emotion to establish a new pattern.

5) The next step is to release the pattern from the cellular memory. This is done by smelling the essential oil, then applying it to the alarm point(s) and the emotional points. To activate an essential oil, place a drop in the palm of your non-dominant hand and rotate it clockwise three times. Then place it on the alarm and emotional points. If you have oil left over, you may wish to apply it to the Release and/or Filter points as described below.

Typical application frequencies are 1, 3, 7, 10, or 18 times per day for 1, 3, or 7 weeks. Different emotions may be treated, one immediately following another. When different oils are required, they may be layered meaning one oil is applied directly on top of or following another. The oils may be applied as close as 15 minutes apart, so you can use them before and after work or at the times when you have a chance to focus on the emotions. If you find you are not able to use the oil as frequently as desired, or need to take some time off to process the emotions, you can extend the length of time the oils are applied.

Release and Filter Points

The Release point, located at the spinal cord at the base of the skull, assists in releasing the emotional pattern. The Filter points located on both sides of the back of the skull are used to filter energies that would pull a person back into the old pattern. These are additional enhancement points that can be used periodically once the essential oil has been applied to the alarm points and the frontal eminences.

Oil Sensitivity

Some oils are strong and may be irritating to sensitive skin, especially on the face and forehead. If you experience drying or burning, dilute the oil by adding V6 or any vegetable oil to the drop in the palm of your hand. If you experience any difficulty with the oils, simply smell the oil and touch the alarm and emotional points, feeling the emotions and saying the statement.

Certain oils like *Lemon* can cause a person to be photosensitive–burning easily in bright sunlight. Use these oils with caution, smelling rather than applying.

Once the oil has been initially applied, feeling the feelings and saying the statement is often effective when using the oil is inconvenient.

The most important element is your intention. Feel the feelings and focus on the statement. There may be times when the statement is unclear. As you work with it, new awarenesses will surface. This is a learning, unfolding process.

Working With Small Children

As a parent, you can apply the oil for the appropriate emotion to the acupuncture alarm points and the emotional points, saying the emotions and the statement. This is particularly effective when both the parent and child are working on the same issue, since children will often act out and reflect what is going on unconsciously for the parent.

The ultimate goal is to teach children to change negative emotions into positive expressions. One of the most common emotions is anger which usually flares when a child doesn't get his or her way. The oil for the emotion of anger is *Purification*. The easiest Liver alarm point to access is on the hands. Applying the oil will often shift the anger within minutes.

For more stubborn or deeply engrained patterns, a physical activity that doesn't hurt anyone such as taking the child outside with you and doing something physical, like kicking clumps of dirt, will shift anger into laughter. The key is both of you need to engage in a silly physical activity. Before you know it, you will both be laughing.

Another common emotion for children is hurt. The oil is *Passion* and the other side is creativity. To provide a physical association, give the child a piece of colored paper and encourage him or her to tear a shape out of the paper like a ball, bell, or flower. Keep the paper shapes in a basket where they can be reviewed. This shows how hurts can be changed into creativity which results in being worthwhile–an important step in building selfesteem.

Helping Others

When emotions surface, like anger for example, start by saying, "I'm feeling anger." Then smell the oil, *Purification*, and apply it to yourself. Say the other side of the emotion which is laughter and state the "way out," "My direction is clear." Then offer to share the oil with those around you. Regardless of what they choose to do, the situation will shift.

You may be aware of underlying emotions that the person you are assisting is unable to address on his/her own. You can use the oil associated with the emotion in a foot massage or over the area of the body where the alarm point is located. The emotions can be stated along with the statement of the "way out." For further enhancement, the oil relating to the dominant emotion(s) can be added to a diffuser and placed by the person's bed.

DISCOVERING THE EMOTION

There are numerous ways of identifying the emotion(s). Since they are interrelated, you may use any one or several because there will be overlapping. Use the entry point that is most prominent at the time.

1. Identify the emotion.

   Go to Emotional Reference and find the emotion.

2. Determine the area of pain, pressure or discomfort in the body.

   Refer to Charts for the body alarm points.

   Then go to Body Reference for the emotion.

   Then go to Emotional Reference.

3. Find the oil. You may have a scent you are particularly attracted to.

   Go to Oils Reference and find the emotion that relates to what is going on in your life.

4. Reflex points on the foot or ear.

   Find the tender spot(s) and the related body alarm point or emotion.

5. Body Type: determine your body type and refer to the related core issues.

   Select the one(s) that have the greatest emotional charge.

6. Dominant traits—show major areas of strengths and challenges.

   Select the one(s) you would like to support.

7. Communicate with your body by hearing what it has to say through meditation, or by asking through more tangible methods such as dowsing, muscle testing or the body movement test.

POINTS OF CONNECTION

Knowing your dominant traits will help you determine which oils will consistently benefit you. Dominant traits are your "points of connection" and will lead you to your greatest area of imbalance. There are 4 traits: mental, emotional, physical and spiritual, two of which will be stronger or dominant. Everyone has a stronger connection with either their mind—Mental, or feelings—Emotional. There will also be a stronger connection between the Spiritual—intuitive, or Physical aspects. The strongest ones are the ones that seem the most real; they are the ones that feel the most comfortable. The other two are present to a greater or lesser degree. How well you have integrated them will determine how familiar they feel to you.

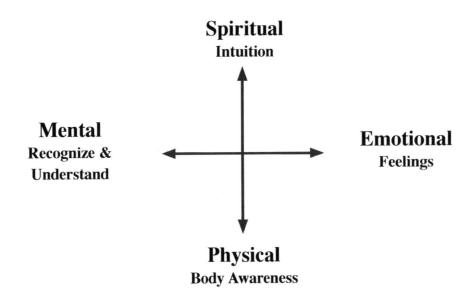

Dominant Trait Combinations

You are born with two dominant or strongest traits. The challenge is to strengthen, integrate and balance the other two with your dominant traits. Once you have identified your dominant traits, look at how they are being expressed in your life. Is there one that is overactive and needs to be relaxed, or is there a weak one that needs to be strengthened? A dominant trait can be overactive, meaning it needs to be relaxed, calmed down or sedated. Sometimes the complimentary trait needs to be strengthened or stimulated. The words and questions on the following two pages are included to help you determine your dominant traits or "points of connection".

"Points of connection" are the areas that you identify with most. The goal is to connect with and integrate the opposite points. The more you have done to develop your recessive trait, the harder it is to distinguish your strongest tendency. *If you have integrated your opposite side, remember back to a time before you made the decision to develop your recessive trait.*

To determine your "points of connection," honestly look at yourself. With both the words and statements, select the set that relates to your basic nature. *Answer according to your feelings, not what you were taught.* Remember, one is not better than another.

MENTAL vs. EMOTIONAL

What sense do you ultimately rely on, mental or emotional? This is often your first impulse, or your strongest influence. When faced with a difficult situation, do you rely most heavily on your ability to think it through logically (mental), or your "gut" feeling on how to handle the situation (emotional)?

The words and statements below are attributes of each sense. Choose the ones that best reflect your basic nature or tendencies.

Think	Feel
Rely on Mind	Rely on Feelings
Logic	Gut Feeling
Focused	Let it Be
To the Point	Expansive
Linear	Random
Peace	Warm Fuzzies
Ambition	Commitment
Passion	Belief
Drive	Action
My initial response is to think first, feel later.	My initial response to situations is to feel first, then think about it.
At home, I respond best to reasonable requests.	At home, I respond best to direct requests.
I tend to approach my feelings and those of others from a detached, analytical point of view.	I tend to become immersed in feelings, both mine and others.
I prefer conversations to be logical, orderly and non-emotional.	I prefer conversations that deal emotionally with issues.
My dominant sense is mental.	My dominant sense is emotional.
MENTAL	**EMOTIONAL**

Are you more Mental or Emotional, or Emotional who doesn't display feelings?

PHYSICAL vs. SPIRITUAL

Do you relate or identify more with your body or your spirit? Are you a spirit with a body or a body with a spirit? If you identify most with your body, your reality is closely associated with your physical body, strength, or physical presence. If you identify most with your spirit, your reality is characterized by intuition and a physical caution. People with a strong spiritual connection often approach unfamiliar situations and physical experiences with caution, while physicals will jump right in.

Select the words you are most attracted to and the statements that best describe your natural tendencies.

Sturdy	Fragile
Ground	Air
Solid	Delicate
Earth	Sky
Literal	Etheral
Scientific	Magical
Anchored	Floating
Visible	Unseen
Environment	Universe
Grounded	Flexible
Tangible	Invisible
Manifestation	Idea
Sensory	Sensitive
Precise	Conceptual
Factual	Intuitive
I prefer life to be orderly and straightforward	I prefer life to occur with a natural ebb & flow.
I prefer to hear a new idea several. times before I try it.	I enjoy trying new ideas or concepts immediately.
I go from the details to the big picture	I go from the big picture to the details.
I am a body with a spirit.	I am a spirit wih a body.
PHYSICAL	**SPIRITUAL**

Is your dominant trait physical or spiritual? Select the one that reflects your basic childhood nature.

DOMINANT TRAITS

One of the ways of determining your core issues is by looking at the emotion stored in the gland, organ, or system that relates to your dominant gland or body type. The 25 body types[6] can be divided into 4 quadrants based on their dominant traits.

PHYSICAL / MENTAL

- Adrenal
- Lymph
- Medulla
- Nervous System
- Spleen
- Stomach
- Thymus

SPIRITUAL / MENTAL

- Balanced
- Brain
- Eye
- Hypothalamus
- Pineal
- Pituitary
- Thalamus
- Thyroid

PHYSICAL / EMOTIONAL

- Blood
- Gallbadder
- Gonadal
- Kidney
- Liver
- Lung
- Pancreas
- Skin

SPIRITUAL / EMOTIONAL

- Heart
- Intestinal

---

[6] *Different Bodies, Different Diets* with the 25 Body Type System™ by Carolyn L. Mein, D.C. 1998

TRAITS

HINT: Each quadrant contains several body types. Some of them will express the extreme of the traits while others will be very close to the opposite traits, making it difficult to feel totally confident in your selection. For example, while both are in the Physical/Mental quadrant, Thymus types relate strongly with the Physical traits, while Lymphs gravitate more toward the Spiritual traits. Lymphs are still Physical, as they will use physical activity to move into a sense of spiritual oneness. As you read through the traits, your type's expression will become clear.

Expressions of the Quadrant

PHYSICAL/MENTAL
The tangible world is reality. They need to see it, touch it, and understand how it works, for it to be real. Physically strong and mentally focused, they can achieve whatever they set out to do.

SPIRITUAL/MENTAL
Ideas, ideals, and concepts are their reality. Figuring out how to synthesize bits of information and insights to express in physical form for the good of mankind is their strength, making them more task-oriented, rather than primarily socially focused.

PHYSICAL/EMOTIONAL
Emotions and physically expressing feelings are their reality, so family and social relationships are their highest priority.

SPIRITUAL/EMOTIONAL
Extremely sensitive in both the spiritual and the emotional traits, these types generally learn to focus on the physical and mental traits early in life to survive. Their power lies in using their strengths.

The challenge and goal for all is to develop and integrate the non-dominant traits or other side. To help us, we attract people whose strengths are different from ours. The traits you are working on are the ones you are developing, rather than the ones you own. While there are two traits, one may be stronger than the other depending on your life focus. For example, a Thyroid man who has focused on the mental aspect of his life may have difficulty identifying with the spiritual side. In this case, he would want to develop his recessive dominant trait as well as the non-dominant ones. Blocked expression most often occurs around the Spiritual and Emotional traits.

INDIVIDUAL BODY TYPE TRAITS

ADRENAL TRAITS
The Adrenal dominant traits are Physical and Mental. There is no sweeter pleasure than success—success in every aspect of life. For it to be real, success has to have a physical expression, like cars, money, recognition, acceptance, the bigger the better. The focus is mental so emotions are secondary. It is easy to ignore or suppress them, until suddenly there is an emotional explosion. The triggering incident is generally unrelated; once the tirade is over, the air is clear—no grudges, residuals, or regrets.

BALANCED TRAITS

The Balanced dominant traits are Spiritual and Mental. The Balanced Body Type thrives on dventureand people are the greatest adventure. Their dominant mental trait provides an intellectual quickness while the Spiritual aspect brings a sensitivity and compassion towards others They love to be on stage as entertaining is a creative, expressive, social adventure.

BLOOD TRAITS

The Blood dominant traits are Physical and Emotional. Harmony is absolutely essential for Blood Body Types. They relate to the world through feeling. So they are constantly aware of their emotions and their perception of others' emotional states. Needing to respect themselves and be respected by others, clearing any disharmony, real or perceived, is a high priority.

BRAIN TRAITS

The Brain dominant traits are Spiritual and Mental. They are happiest when they have a direction. With a strong mental trait, gathering information is easy, and their intuitive spiritual side fills in the gaps. Having a direction allows them to feel safe and gives them a purpose in taking what they have collected out into the world. Getting out into the world opens them to growth by exposing them to physical and emotional experiences.

EYE TRAITS

The Eye dominant traits are Spiritual and Mental. Eyes need to make a difference for their lives to have meaning. Visionaries, they see the way things could be, the way they are and what needs to happen to make the change. Making a difference in someone else's life is an effective way of bringing their vision into physical reality. Their sensitive Spiritual aspect allows them to observe without judgment and makes them aware of the effect that simply releasing negative emotions has on people. With their strength being Mental, it is easy to ignore or repress unpleasant emotions, even to the point of closing off their vision if they feel too overwhelmed.

GALLBLADDER TRAITS

The Gallbladder dominant traits are Physical and Emotional. While emotional, Gallbladders tend to keep their feelings to themselves and are most fulfilled when they can physically express their love for those around them by being useful. Physical activity helps them sort things out and focus their emotions. Their solid, physical strength is reflected in their dependable, consistent nature.

GONADAL TRAITS

The Gonadal dominant traits are Physical and Emotional. Being playful provides the ideal environment to express the full range of the positive side of their emotions with those they love. Being highly verbal and sensitive to others' emotions often leads to their own emotional volatility. Gonadals are motivated by beauty, which makes it important to look good, and can even include a strong, proud, macho image. Their strength lies in seeing beauty and bringing out the beauty of others. True inner beauty is most readily accessed when being playful.

HEART TRAITS

The Heart dominant traits are Spiritual and Emotional. Highly aware of and sensitive to the emotional states of those around them, Hearts feel best when their environment is at peace. Disharmony makes them so uncomfortable, that they will do or say something to shift the energy. When that isn't effective or appropriate, they will physically move out of the space and create a new space, inviting others to move into their energy.

HYPOTHALAMUS TRAITS

The Hypothalamus dominant traits are Spiritual and Mental. A challenge provides the focus necessary for the Hypothalamus to go to the depths, immersing themselves in an endeavor which ultimately develops another trait of themselves to share with their world. Their strong analytical mind and sensitive intuition allows them to excel in the creation of companies, financial empires, or a way of life to benefit first themselves, then mankind.

INTESTINAL TRAITS

The Intestinal dominant traits are Spiritual and Emotional. Expansion is absolutely essential. If Intestinals do not expand mentally or emotionally, they will expand physically. Restriction motivates them to change, forcing them out of an untenable situation into an unknown physical, mental world. It is here where they can genuinely expand, taking in new experiences and creating an environment which is truly peace on earth.

KIDNEY TRAITS

The Kidney dominant traits are Physical and Emotional. Kidneys are happiest when they can be flexible—when they have choices and can explore new options. Once they have accomplished something, and moved beyond their perceived limitations, they relax and enjoy those around them until the next challenge arises. To feel fulfilled, the challenges need to be different and involve people, allowing for greater flexibility and growth.

LIVER TRAITS

The Liver dominant traits are Physical and Emotional. Livers are excellent teachers. Emotionally based, supporting or being supported by people around them provides the motivation to learn what life presents. Livers excel when they are uniting life, putting things together so they flow, passing the wisdom gained by one generation on to the next.

LUNG TRAITS

The Lung dominant traits are Physical and Emotional. Nurturing, either being nurtured or nurturing someone else, provides Lungs with the greatest sense of fulfillment. Emotionally sensitive, the tendency is to project a hard outer shell, or shut down and withdraw when feeling powerless or inadequate. The need for self-expression motivates them to access their creativity which is often linked to music or physical ways of nurturing those around them.

LYMPH TRAITS

The Lymph dominant traits are Physical and Mental. Excitement keeps Lymphs moving, active and alive. Without physical or mental stimulation, they become depressed which in turn brings emotional pain to the surface and motivates them to move out of their depressed state. Mentally quick and alert, learning provides a sense of fulfillment. Physically based, health and physical attractiveness are a high priority.

MEDULLA TRAITS

The Medulla dominant traits are Physical and Mental. Medullas thrive when they are appreciated. Their patience and systematic, logical approach make them excellent teachers. The appreciation of their students keeps them motivated, while their strong mental focus and fear of failure keeps them consistently alert and up to date in their field.

NERVOUS SYSTEM TRAITS

The Nervous System dominant traits are Physical and Mental. Nothing provides a greater sense of satisfaction than listening to others. Practical and efficient, they excel when they use their strong mental abilities to gather information and share it with others according to their needs and desires, connecting people with information.

PANCREAS TRAITS

The Pancreas dominant traits are Physical and Emotional. Pancreas Types are truly fulfilled when they feel joy and can share their joy with others. Being emotionally based, there is often a feeling of insecurity when they compare themselves to their mentally based friends which motivates them to develop their mental side. However, it's the emotional energy that keeps an organization running and joy that keeps it humming.

PINEAL TRAITS

The Pineal dominant traits are Spiritual and Mental. Pineals need to have a sense of freedom to feel fulfilled. Ultimate freedom comes from the spiritual aspect and manifests as self-realization. Intuition is an expression of the Spiritual and one of the gifts of self-realization. Mentally quick and alert, the challenge is to connect with the heart and integrate the emotions. True freedom is only experienced when negative or self-limiting emotional patterns have been cleared.

PITUITARY TRAITS

The Pituitary dominant traits are Spiritual and Mental. The ultimate rewarding experience for Pituitary Types is feeling happy. Children learn more in the first four years of their lives than the total of everything learned thereafter. With their dominant spiritual connection, Pituitaries are able to maintain their wide eyed innocence and childlike openness throughout their lives. Their strong mental acuity allows them to take what they learn and use it to assist others so they too can feel happy.

SKIN TRAITS

The Skin dominant traits are Physical and Emotional. There is no greater thrill than discovery, and the most thrilling discoveries are those that emotionally benefit themselves and those around them. Being highly visual, Skins like to express their discoveries in a physical, tangible form, preferably something that feels good. Acutely feeling others' emotions, they like to make others feel good and love being touched.

SPLEEN TRAITS

The Spleen dominant traits are Physical and Mental. They are happiest when they are feeling secure. Being physical, security needs to be tangible, like a big house, money in the bank, a viable project and/or having someone physically present. With their strong mental focus, they are excellent organizers and have the tenacity to see that even huge events come out right.

STOMACH TRAITS

The Stomach dominant traits are Physical and Mental. Stomachs love a challenge–any challenge will do, as their ultimate sense of fulfillment comes from accomplishment. Their strong mental focus and the physical power behind it makes them extremely passionate about whatever challenge happens to be within their focus. Their desire to please opens the door for emotional sensitivity. Connecting with their spiritual side focuses their tremendous mental and physical energy.

THALAMUS TRAITS

The Thalamus dominant traits are Spiritual and Mental. The Thalamus type is fulfilled by being, rather than doing. Their greatest satisfaction comes from being effective, or being worthwhile, making their expression more internal than external. With a strong mental sense, they love to gather information and file it away for future reference, so research is second nature to them. Their dominant spiritual trait is reflected in their strong auditory sense, making them highly responsive to music and sensitive to sound.

THYMUS TRAITS

The Thymus dominant traits are Physical and Mental. The Thymus Body Type is fulfilled by meeting a personal challenge. Being extremely protective of their own, the challenge is often initiated by physical pain. Physically and mentally oriented, they can be quite pragmatic in their approach to life. The challenge is to integrate the spiritual and emotional traits, moving from judgment to unconditional love and acceptance–perfection in this lifetime.

THYROID TRAITS

The Thyroid dominant traits are Spiritual and Mental. For an activity to be rewarding, it needs to be worthwhile, meaning it makes a worthwhile contribution to someone or humanity in general. At home in their heads, Thyroids' contributions are to take the information they have gathered from the spiritual and mental realms and express it in ways that help humanity. By bridging the gap between the head and heart, they physically express the spiritual. To fulfill their destiny, Thyroids need to share their discoveries.

THE 25 BODY TYPE SYSTEM™

There are 25 different body types with unique nutritional and exercise needs – and personality profiles – as determined by the dominant gland, organ or system of your body.

You can now determine your body type using the online test found at:

www.bodytype.com

Select "Women's Test" or "Men's Test"

CORE EMOTIONAL ISSUES

While we all have all the emotional patterns, some are more of an issue for some of us than others. Each body type has certain lessons or challenges that are characteristically challenging for that type. The following list is the most common core emotional issues for each body type.

BODY TYPE	EMOTION	BODY TYPE	EMOTION
Adrenal	Conflict, Failure, Abandonment, Facing the World	Lymph	(Being) Left Behind, Identity
Balanced	Control, Rejection, F—You	Medulla	Restriction, Failure
Blood	Disharmony, Conflict, Crushed, Trapped	Nervous System	Victim, Anger, Control, F—You
Brain	Abandonment, Wrong Addiction, Abuse, Control, Inferiority, Failure	Pancreas	Wrong, Betrayal, Letting go
Eye	Emotions, F—You, Overwhelmed	Pineal	Control, Unknown, Restriction
Gallbladder	Past (Fear of repeating), Frustration, Resentment, Letting Go	Pituitary	Aloneness, Abandonment, Wisdom, Restriction
Gonadal	Identity, Repression, Not good Enough	Skin	Criticism, Abandonment
Heart	Loneliness, Not Good Enough, Worry	Spleen	Guilt, Abandonment, Wrong
Hypothalamus	Shame, Fear, Betrayal	Stomach	Abandonment, Control, Victim, Conflict, Inferiority, Stubborn
Intestinal	Abandonment, Not Good Enough, Rejection, Despair, Criticism	Thalamus	Dependence, Failure
Kidney	Love, Fear, Misunderstood	Thymus	Anger, Failure, Losing, Abandonment, Wrong, Inferiority
Liver	Anger, Rejection, Failure	Thyroid	Sadness, Injustice, Speaking out, Failure, Misunderstood
Lung	Rejection, Abandonment, Stubborn		

FOUR TRAITS

Once you have determined whether your dominant sense is mental or emotional, you can look at how it is being expressed. Is your mind too rigid or controlling, dominating your other senses? If so, *Peace & Calming*[7] can help relax your mind. You may also want to use *Joy*[7] to enhance and support your emotions.

Are you too emotional? *Sandalwood*[7] helps to calm overactive emotions. *Clarity*[7] helps to support the mind and bring about mental clarity.

The better you understand the various aspects of yourself, the easier it is to accept yourself, develop, and integrate your other side. Knowing your body type[8] and reading your psychological profile will provide more insights. The body type profile[8] is designed to provide a concise, practical guide to understanding your basic traits, motivation, and the best ways to express your strengths. Determining your two dominant traits will allow you to determine your body type and the related core emotional issues.

The four traits – physical, emotional, mental and spiritual – represent our four bodies. Imbalance in any area is the result of energy being

> too high — overactive, hyper or

> too low — underactive, exhausted, or depleted.

Harmony is a state of balance. Balance can be achieved by determining

> which system is out of balance or stressed

> and whether it is over or underactive

The following oils have generally been found to be highly effective. You'll want to select the oil that will balance the area that needs the most attention.

---

[7] Oil Blends by Young Living Essential Oils™

[8] *Different Bodies, Different Diets* with the 25 Body Type System™ by Carolyn Mein

HARMONIZING EMOTIONS

PHYSICAL

- **Valor** enhances physical strengh. Apply to feet.

  Physical tension is due to the physical body being overactive and this oil helps to release physical focus.

  For added benefit: have 2 people apply the oil with 1 person at the feet and the other at the shoulders, applying the oil to C7 and on the top of the shoulders (nerve points).

- **Immupower** aids in supporting the immune system and is especially helpful when there is a physical illness.

EMOTIONAL

- **Joy** helps to change depression into a positive state.

  Brings in positive emotional qualities and is beneficial in clearing anxiety and grief.

- **Sandalwood** helps when emotions are overactive. Apply to big toes, temples, and base of spine.

- **SARA** helps to clear emotional trauma, allowing one to move from emotional turmoil to mental clarity.

MENTAL

- **Clarity** helps when there is a lack of mental clarity or the brain is underactive.

- **Peace & Calming** is used when the mental aspect becomes overactive.

SPIRITUAL

- **Frankincense** stimulates & elevates the mind.

- **Rose** increases spiritual focus.

- **White Angelica** is particularly good for protection.

- **Awaken** balances mental states & awakens inner knowing.

- **3 Wise Men** promotes grounding & releases deep-seated trauma.

CLEANSING AND MAINTAINING YOUR ENERGY FIELD

Sea Salt

If you are a sensitive person, work with or are around a lot of people, there is a tendency to "pick up" energy from others and hold it in your energy field. Adding sea salt to the bath, or using it like soap in the shower cleanses the emotional body. When using salt in the shower, keep it in a plastic cup, get wet and apply the salt like soap particularly to the chest and solar plexus. It removes dead cells making your skin soft. Use the fine plain sea salt found in bulk in health food stores. The two areas to emphasize are the solar plexus and chest. Using sea salt is particularly helpful when a person is going through his or her own emotional release or is around anyone else who is, and for many, this is generally most of the time.

Essential Oils

The oil blend *White Angelica* can also be used to clear your energy field or aura, in addition to serving as a protection from bombardment from negative energy.

To cleanse your energy field, put a drop or two of *White Angelica* in the palm of your hand. Rub your hands together three times clockwise to activate it. Put your fingertips together above your head. Then bring your hands down along the sides of your body. You may also want to run your hands down the front and back of your body. Since your energy field is larger then your physical body, holding your hands several inches away from your body allows you to quickly clear your energy field.

White Angelica can be placed on the top of the head, sternum (chest bone), top of the shoulders and back of the head near the neck as protection when you are going into a room full of people. If you are particularly sensitive to other people's energies, using *White Angelica* can prevent your picking up their emotional energies and carrying these energies home with you.

This is particularly helpful in allowing you to maintain you own energy and preventing you from being drained when you are at work, in a class, or a demanding corporate meeting.

Clearing your energy field with *White Angelica* can easily be shared with your office staff. It is quick and generally produces immediate, noticeable, positive shifts especially in sensitive individuals.

Peace and Calming is an excellent oil to use on the wrists and top of the shoulders, (as well as the ways listed above) when someone is upset or agitated. It is exceptionally effective for crying babies, young children, and animals.

Center and Balance

Ken Page, in his book, ***The Way It Works***, describes a simple clearing technique that allows you to center and balance your energy. This technique takes less than 30 seconds and ideally should be done when you are alone three or more times a day, in complete privacy, where you basically have nothing else to do but just be. For many of us, the only time this occurs is when we are in the bathroom.

"Whether you are sitting or standing, do the following: using your intent and focus, bring your hands up over your head and as you relieve yourself, simply think 'clear'. As you think 'clear', bring your hands down the front midline of your body. Next, bring yourself into your own space. Do this by simply pulling yourself in, just using your conscious intent and focus. A very easy way to do this is to extend your arms out from your body and focus on the thought that you are now going to pull yourself in. To bring your energetic field in, slowly move your outstretched arms towards your body. Finish by resting your hands over your solar plexus. Now take another 5 to 10 seconds to just be in your space, be in the moment and love yourself."[9]

Maintenance

To determine which oils to use, you may want to tune into the energy of the day. Is there an aspect that needs to be supported or enhanced? You can check to see how are you feeling to determine if you need more support in one area. Once you have cleared the specific emotions you are aware of, your choices will probably come from the Four Traits.

[9] *The Way it Works,* p.28, by Ken Page, 1997

GUIDE TO THE REFERENCES

Emotional Reference

The easiest place to start is to go to the emotion you are most aware of or are currently feeling.

While most of the emotions listed are negative, there are a few that are positive. Obviously, we want to clear the negative and enhance the positive emotions. When there is a positive emotion listed, like love, it refers to the negative emotion around love, like fear of not being loved or being lovable. It can also relate to the fear to love. The oils are adaptagens, meaning they have the ability to balance the emotion, whether it is over or underactive.

Oils Reference

Once you have identified a particular emotion, you may wish to work with related emotions. There is often a relationship between the emotions that require the same oil. You may be attracted to a specific oil and want to know the emotion associated with it.

Body Reference

Look down the list until you find the organ, gland or system that is stressed or where you know you have difficulty. Now that you have found the corresponding emotion, turn to the Emotional Reference.

One way to locate emotions similar to the ones you are experiencing is to look for other related organs or systems. For example, ears are associated with hearing, the eustachian tubes with fear of hearing the truth, and the external ear with fear of incongruency. These can be accessed by related organs through the Body Reference, the Body Alarm Point Reference by physical location of the organs, or through the Emotional Reference by related emotions.

Location of Body Alarm Points

You may not be aware of any emotion, but feel pain or discomfort in your body. Go to the charts, locate the pain and refer to the Body Reference for the associated emotion.

You may work on several emotions simultaneously or give yourself more time to process. When working with a chronic problem, the frequency of use and area of application can change. You'll want to be aware when your body shifts. Simple ways of communicating with your body are through the use of muscle testing. Muscle testing is explained in the last chapter.

You can use the oils to clear specific emotional patterns, or use them simply on an as needed basis. Once you have cleared a pattern, you may be drawn to a periodic "refresher". You may use only the oils you are drawn to with frequency varying from as little as once to multiple uses over an extended period of time. Frequency may vary from one day to another, as can the need for different oils for related emotions assoicated with the same symptom.

References

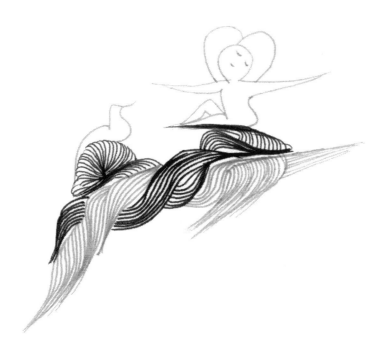

EMOTIONAL REFERENCE

Emotions, the Other Side of the Emotion and the Lesson or "Way Out"

Releasing an emotional pattern that limits you requires understanding the issue and how it affects your life. In other words, understanding why you are experiencing this problem, what you could experience instead, and what you need to do to change. Changing a pattern is like erasing a groove, the deeper it is embedded, the longer you need to erase. For some emotions you may only need to bring them into your awareness to release them. Other more deep rooted emotions will require more time and attention.

All unpleasant emotions are fear-based. The following list of emotions consist of negative feelings or the fear of not experiencing a positive feeling such as love, meaning fear of not being loved or lovable. It could also be fear to love.

EMOTION	OTHER SIDE	WAY OUT	OIL	ALARM POINT	CHART
ABANDONMENT *(Fear of)*	At-one-ment	*I embrace all of life's experiences*	Lavender	Small Intestine	E,F,G,H
ABUNDANCE	Scarcity	*I am in alignment with universal flow*	Abundance	Laryngeal Prominence	A,C
ABUSE *(All/Any)*	Nurtured	*I deserve to be loved*	SARA	Cellular Memory	D,H
ACCEPTANCE	Rejection	*I can be accepted*	SARA	Emotional Point	A
ADDICTION	Freedom	*I am wanted and loveable*	Peace & Calming	Brain	A,B,E,G,H
ADRENAL EXHAUSTION	Strength	*I am complete*	Nutmeg or En-R-Gee	Adrenal	D,G,H
AGGRESSION	Respect	*I love*	Valor	Adrenal Cortex	D
AGITATED	Tranquility	*I am centered*	Rosewood	Blood Pressure	E
ALONE *(Being)*	United	*Be all here*	Purification	Staph	B
ALONENESS	Acceptance of all that is	*I embrace*	Aroma Life	Heart Protector	D
ALOOF	Engaged	*I connect with source*	Northern Lights Black Spruce	Heart Protector	D
AMBIVALENCE	Engaged	*I care*	Celery Seed	Hippocampus	A,C
ANGER	Laughter	*My direction is clear*	Purification	Liver	C,D,G,H

EMOTION	OTHER SIDE	WAY OUT	OIL	ALARM POINT	CHART
ANGUISH	Ecstacy	*I am willing to accept the truth*	Palo Santo	Heart	B,G,H
ANNIHILATION	*See Obliteration*				
ANNOYANCE	Happy	*I relax*	Highest Potential	Courage	E
ANXIETY	Confidence	*Peace, be still*	Joy	Capillary	D
APATHY	Enthusiasm	*I am aware*	Brain Power	Hippocampus	A,C
APPROVAL	*See Rejection*				
ARGUMENTIVENESS	Peace	*I am fair*	Peace & Calming	Thyroid	A,C,G,H
ARROGANCE	*See Unknown*				
ATTACHMENT	Connection	*I hold the vision*	Envision	Vision	B
ATTACK	*See Fear of Losing*				
AUTHORITY (*Rebelling against or resentment of*)	Clarity	*I see with clarity*	JuvaFlex or Birch	Bone	F
BAD (*Feeling*)	Change	*I am creating*	Gathering	Kidney	D,G,H
BALANCED	*See Control*				
BELONG (*Don't*)	*See Don't Belong*				
BEATING SELF UP	*See Punishment*				
BELITTLED	Recognized	*I see myself*	Lime	Vision	B
BETTER THAN, LESS THAN	*See Inferiority* and/or *Unworthy, Less Than*				
BETRAYAL (*Fear of*)	Trust	*I have the courage to accept the truth*	Forgiveness	Pancreas	C,G,H
BITTERNESS	*See Past*				

EMOTION	OTHER SIDE	WAY OUT	OIL	ALARM POINT	CHART
BLACK HOLE *(Being in a)*	Clarity	*I am surrounded and protected*	Pepper, Black	Temporal Bone, Mastoid Portion	B
BLAME	Balance	*I understand*	JuvaFlex	Toxic	E
BLINDNESS	Illumination	*I breathe with certainty*	Hope	Eye Lymph	A
BLINDSIDED	Aware	*I am alert*	Rosewood	Temporal Bone, Mastoid Portion	B
BONDAGE *(Fear of)*	Freedom	*I like who I am*	Eucalyptus Globulus	Parotid	B
BOREDOM	Direction	*I am in alignment*	Grounding	Parasites	D
BRAIN FOG	Unity	*I come together*	Brain Power or GeneYus	Roof of mouth *(suck thumb)*	
CAN'T	Can	*I accept all that I am*	Transformation	Virus	D,E,H
CELLULAR MEMORY *(Clearing)*	Freedom	*I release the past*	Inner Child	DNA	B
CHAOS	*See Obliteration*				
CHANGE *(Resistance to)*	Steady	*I learn from all of life's experiences*	Present Time	Rectum	E,G
CHEATED	*See Deprived*				
CHOKED	Empowered	*I am renewed and aligned*	Longevity	Vibration	D
CLAUSTROPHOBIA	*See Confined*				
CO-DEPENDENCY	Interdependency	*Life supports me*	Sandalwood	Emotional Integration	A,B,E
COMMITMENT	Manifestation	*I am free*	Transformation	Ego	E
COMPETITIVENESS	Growth	*I excel*	Dream Catcher	Lymph Valves	C
COMPLAISANCE	Responsible	*I transform*	Exodus II	Magic	C
COMPLETION *(Fear of)*	Development	*I am conscientious*	Oregano or Marjoram	Anterior Fontanel	B

EMOTION	OTHER SIDE	WAY OUT	OIL	ALARM POINT	CHART
COMPROMISING (Self)	Truth	*I express truth*	Sacred Mountain	Soul	B,F
CONCEIT	Meekness	*I know who I am*	Cedarwood	Hypothalamus 6th Chakra	A,E
CONFINED	Freedom	*I allow myself to see*	Envison	Intuitive	E
CONFLICT (Fear of)	Peace	*I am at peace*	Valor	Adrenal Cortex	D
CONFRONTATION	*See Conflict*				
CONFUSION	Focus	*I am centered and focused*	Magnify Your Purpose	Integration @ L3	F
CONNECTING INTERDIMENSIONALLY	Wholeness	*I am complete*	Awaken	Sacral Door	F
CONNECTION	*See Isolation*				
CONSCIOUSNESS (Shifting)	Taking Personal Responsibility	*I am changing*	Laurus Nobilis *or* White Angelica	Aorta	A,C
CONSEQUENCES	*See Guilt*				
CONTROLLING BY ATTACKING	Flexible	*I am safe*	Common Sense	Ileum	E
CONTROL (Fear of losing)	Balance	*I am content and blessed*	Peace & Calming	Stomach	C,E,G,H
COPE (Inability to)	Live	*I come from my strength*	Valor	White Blood Cells	F
CRISIS	Relieved	*I am divinely guided*	White Angelica	Esophagus	E,G
CRITICISM	Unconditional love and acceptance	*I receive*	Lavender	Skin	F
CRUSHED	Expand	*I rise*	Harmony	Blood	C
CYNICISM	Understanding	*I accept the truth*	Transformation	Small Intestine	E,F,G,H
DEATH/LIVING (Fear of)	Life	*I am a success*	Helichrysum	Arteries	B,D
DECEIVED	Vision	*I see clearly*	Ravensara	Eye/Brain on Occipit	B,F

EMOTION	OTHER SIDE	WAY OUT	OIL	ALARM POINT	CHART
DEFEATED	Honored	*Life supports me*	Tsuga	CNS / Lymph	A,B,C
DEFENSELESS	Powerful	*I am powerful*	Goldenrod	Adrenal Cortex	D
DEFENSIVENESS	Receptive	*I am open*	Valor	Stomach	C,E,G,H
DEFIANCE	*See "F-You"*				
DEGRADED	Nurtured	*I assert myself*	Pine	White Blood Cells	F
DEJECTION	Spontaneous joy	*I release limitation*	Release	Pleura	C
DENIAL	Acceptance	*I acknowledge*	Endoflex	Vision	B
DEPENDENCE (*Fear of*)	Freedom	*I am self-sufficient*	Peppermint	Thalamus	A,B,E
DEPENDENT	Steadfast	*I am determined*	Cassia	Will @ C5	B
DEPLETION	Rejuvenated	*I take care of myself*	RC	Lymphatic Congestion	C
*DEPRESSION	Alive	*I am glad I am alive*	Peace & Calming	Depression	B,F
DEPRIVED	Fulfilled	*I am satisfied*	JuvaFlex or Birch	Joints & Cartilage	E
DERAILED	*See Limbo*				
DESERTION	Inner Guidance	*I am totally connected*	Inner Child	RNA	B
DESERVE	*See Guilt*				
DESPAIR	Dignity	*I am open to guidance*	3 Wise Men	Diaphragm	C,G
*DETACHMENT (*Fear of*)	Sustained	*I can stand alone*	Lemon	Spinal Cord	B,F,H

---

* *Depression is often repression; look for underlying emotion.*

* *Detachment — refers to not being connected with inner strength; Sustained — being sustained by a Higher Power; I can stand alone — detaching the illusion that the outside world sustains you.*

EMOTION	OTHER SIDE	WAY OUT	OIL	ALARM POINT	CHART
DEVASTATED	See Not Good Enough				
DEVOID	See Confusion				
DIABOLICAL DISORIENTATION	Divinely Protected	I am divinely protected	Elemi	3rd Eye	A,E
DIFFERENT	Real	I embrace consciousness	Thieves	Mold	D
DIFFICULTY	Knowing	I move with life	Legacy or Myrrh	PSIS	F
DIRECTION (Lack of)	See Procrastination				
DISAPPOINTMENT	Freedom	I trust my vision	Joy	Bronchial	C,G
DISASSOCIATION	Integrated	I am connected	German Chamomile	Soul (C2)	B,F
DISCARDED	See Abandonment				
DISCERNMENT	See Judgement				
DISCOMBOBULATED	See Obliteration				
DISCONNECTED	Secure	I am connected	Marjoram	Umbilicus/Yeast	C,D
DISCOURAGED	See Overwhelmed				
DISEMPOWERED	Respect	I am true to myself	Melaleuca Ericifolia (Rosalina) or Tea Tree	C1	B,F
DISEMPOWERMENT	See Sorcery				
DISGUST	Empowerment	I see the purpose	Australian Blue	Bronchial	C,G
DISHARMONY	Balance	I am centered	White Angelica	Parathyroid	A,B,D,G,H
DISHONESTY	Honesty	I am true to myself	Believe	Spleen	D,G,H

EMOTION	OTHER SIDE	WAY OUT	OIL	ALARM POINT	CHART
DISILLUSIONED	Substance	*I see the reality*	Di-Gize or Di-Tone	Appendix	D,H
DISINTEGRATED	Unity	*I am whole*	Rose	Virus	D,E,H
DISOWNED	*See Enslaved*				
DISRESPECT	Respect	*I am free of insecurity*	Cypress	Veins	D
DISSATISFACTION	Gratitude	*I open my heart*	Ledum	Magic	C
DISTORTION	Innocence	*I am free to let life unfold*	Inner Child	Innocence	A,B
DISTRESS	Grateful	*I accept*	Grapefruit	Heart Strings	D
DISTRUST	Integrity	*I honor truth*	Forgiveness	Uterus/Prostate	C
DIZZINESS (or **Vertigo***)	Directed	*I take back my movement*	Frankincense	Middle Ear	B
DOMINEERING or DOMINATION	*See Control*				
DON'T BELONG	Acceptance	*I value myself*	Acceptance	Solar Plexus	D,G
DON'T KNOW WHERE TO TURN	*See Despair*				
DON'T WANT TO	*See Rebellion*				
DON'T WANT TO MISS ANYTHING	*See Abandonment* and/or *Deprived* and/or *Left Behind*				
DOOMED	Freed	*I forgive*	Exodus II	Solar Plexus	D,G
DOUBT	*See Survival*				
DRAINED	Complete	*I am open to source*	Ylang Ylang	Heart Strings	D
DREAD	Passion	*I embrace my essence*	Sandalwood *or* Live w/ Passion	Arteries	B,D

---

* *Vertigo – Losing balance, spinning.*

EMOTION	OTHER SIDE	WAY OUT	OIL	ALARM POINT	CHART
EMBARRASSED	Embrace	*I am not alone*	Acceptance	Hypothalamus	A,E
EMOTIONAL BOUNDARIES	*See Compromising Self*				
EMOTIONS *(Fear of)*	Feeling	*I let go and allow*	PanAway	Fascia	E,H
EMOTIONS, SUPPRESSED	Protected	*It is safe to remember*	Eucalyptus Blue	Eye/Brain on Occipit	B,F
EMOTIONS, SWALLOWED	Movement	*I raise my awareness*	Hyssop	Epiglottis	A,B,D
EMPTINESS *(Feeling of)vt*	Full	*I am complete*	Lemon	Breast	D,E
ENGULFMENT	*See Identity*				
ENSLAVED	Release	*I am released*	Gathering	Meninges	B,F
ENTITLEMENT	Realistic	*I can do it*	Lemon	Parathyroid	A,B,D,G,H
ENVY	*See Lack*				
ERRATIC ENERGY	Harmony	*I am centered*	Inner Child	Duodenum	E
ESTRANGED	Connected	*I am open*	Spikenard *or* Melissa	Heart Strings	D
EXHAUSTION	Energy	*I nurture myself*	PanAway	Muscle	F
EXPANSION	Contraction	*I allow change*	Awaken	Soul Integration	B
EXPECTATIONS	Appreciating	*I am complete within myself*	SARA	Bladder 2nd Chakra	C,E,G,H
"F-YOU"	Detachment	*I stand in my power*	Frankincense	Ego	E,H
FACING THE WORLD *(Fear of)*	Embracing the world	*I am safe*	Myrrh	Adrenal	D,G,H
FAILURE	Unfoldment	*I accept growth*	Peppermint	Thymus	A,C

EMOTION	OTHER SIDE	WAY OUT	OIL	ALARM POINT	CHART
FAITH *(Lack of)*	Knowingness	*I am connected with Spirit*	Sandalwood	3rd Eye	A,E
FATIGUE	Ignited	*I am aligned*	Inspiration	Life Force	F
FEAR	Awareness / Faith *(Face it)*	*I face the unknown*	Sandalwood	3rd Eye	A,E
FLUSTERED	Present	*I am present*	Present Time	Periosteum	E,F
FOCUS *(Lack of)*	*See Confusion*				
FRIGHTENED	Peaceful	*I listen*	RutaVaLa	Ego	E,H
FROZEN	Vital	*I move with ease*	Eucalyptus Blue	Bladder	C,E,G,H
FRUSTRATION	Accomplishment	*I move beyond my limitations*	Lemon	Common Bile Duct	C,H
FULFILLMENT	*See Unfulfilled*				
FUTILITY	*See Powerless*				
FUTURE	*See Unknown*				
GET EVEN	Accomplishment	*I express my potential*	Highest Potential	Thyroid	A,C,G,H
GIVING UP – or ***What's the point?*** or ***Going through the emotions*** or ***Who cares?***	*See Not Good Enough* and/or *Unimportant*				
GIVING YOUR POWER AWAY	*See Panic* and/or *Powerless*				
GOING FORWARD	*See Fear* and/or *Unknown*				
GREED	Giving	*I am enough*	White Angelica	Heart Constrictor 4th Chakra	C
GRIEF	Happy	*Change brings growth*	Joy	Adenoids	A,B,D

EMOTION	OTHER SIDE	WAY OUT	OIL	ALARM POINT	CHART
GRUDGE	See Resentment				
GUILT	Deserve (Get what you)	I learn from all of life's experiences	Clarity	Spleen	D,G,H
HATE or HATRED	Forgiveness	I am forgiven	Ledum	Hepatic Duct	E
HEARING (Fear of)	Acknowledgment	I have the strength to face reality	Sacred Mountain	Ears, Inner	B,H
HELPLESS	See Overwhelmed and/or Powerless				
HOLDING BACK (Universal flow)	Clear channel	I am perfect timing	Release	Trachea	A,B,C
HOMELESSNESS	See Abandonment				
HOPELESSNESS	Hopeful	There is a way out	Awaken	Bone Marrow	D
HOSTILITY	Harmony	I value life	Harmony	Harmony	F
HUMILIATION	Honor	I manifest divine qualities	Magnify Your Purpose	Skin	F
HURT	Creativity	I am worthwhile	Live with Passion	Creativity	F
HYPERVIGILANCE	See Paranoid				
HYSTERICAL	See Anxiety				
IDENTITY (Loss of)	Purpose	I am in touch with my purpose	Release	Uterus/Prostate	C
IGNORED (Being)	Self-acknowledgment	I am one with all	Harmony	Strep	A,C
ILLUSION	Clarity	I see clearly	Present Time	Virus	D,E,H
IMPATIENCE	Adaptability	I am flexible	Melrose	Immune	C
INADAPTABILITY	See Impatience				

EMOTION	OTHER SIDE	WAY OUT	OIL	ALARM POINT	CHART
INADEQUATE	Empowered	*I am divinely directed*	White Fir *or* Idaho Balsam Fir	GV-20	B
INCAPACITATED	Empowered	*I am centered*	Hinoki	Bone-Center of Sacrum	F
INCOMPETENCE	*See Expectations*				
INCOMPLETION	Progress	*I know my destiny*	Western *or* Canadian Red Cedar *or* Cedarwood	Will @ C-5	B
INCONGRUENCY	Real	*I see the larger picture*	Joy	Ears, External	B
INCONSISTENCY	Consistency	*I can trust myself*	Aroma Siez	Unconscious	B,D
INDECISIVENESS	Focus	*I have clarity*	Peace & Calming	Higher Will @ C-3	B,F
INERTIA	Courage	*I am propelled forward*	Motivation	Courage	E
INFERIORITY	Conscientious	*I express my value*	3 Wise Men	Ileocecal Valve	A,E,G
INJURY	Healing	*I learn*	Melrose	Periosteum	E,F
INJUSTICE (Not fair)	Resolution	*I accept the truth*	Sacred Mountain	Thyroid	A,C,G,H
INSECURITY (Insecure)	Success	*I learn from all life's experiences*	Acceptance	Ileum	E
INSULTED	Humility	*I detach*	Ocotea	Ego	E,H
INTEGRATION	*See Disintegrated*				
INTEGRITY, LACK OF	Honesty	*I am trustworthy*	Helichrysum	Brain	A,B,E,G,H
INTIMACY (Fear of)	Trust	*I am in tune with my direction*	Rose	Heart Center	E
INTIMIDATED	Confident	*I am stable*	Blue Tansy *or* Idaho Tansy	Hormone	A,E

EMOTION	OTHER SIDE	WAY OUT	OIL	ALARM POINT	CHART
INTOLERANCE (General)	Reasonable	*I am tolerant*	Clary Sage	Toxic	E
IRRESPONSIBLE	Acknowledgement	*I face reality and am responsible for my success*	Helichrysum	Eustachian Tubes	B,G
IRRITATION	Bliss	*Bliss runs through me*	Cinnamon Bark	Head of Pancreas	C,E
ISOLATION	Connection	*I am integrated*	En-R-Gee	Yeast/Umbilicus	C,D
JEALOUSY	*See Left Behind*				
JUDGEMENT	Regard	*I am discerning*	Joy	Solar Plexus	D,G
LACK	Faith	*I trust I can change*	Ginger	Peyer's Patches	D
LASHING OUT	Discretion	*Truth comes through me*	Clove	Tongue	B
LAZY	Initiative	*I am motivated*	Spearmint	Pancreatic Duct	E
LEFT BEHIND	Move	*I am free to move forward*	Lemon	Lymph	C
LESS THAN, BEING	Sharing	*I am appropriate*	Humility	Medulla	B,F
LETTING GO	Happiness	*Let go and let God* or *Let go and let live*	Sage	Bladder	C,E,G,H
LIES	Truth	*Wisdom*	Copaiba	Spinal Cord	B,F
LIFE (Suppression of)	Contact	*I regenerate*	Myrtle	Chi	E
LIFELESS	Exist	*I exist*	RutaVaLa	Hara midway b/t Ego & Solar Plexus	D
LIMBO	Trust	*I am divinely guided*	Palo Santo	3rd Eye	A,E
LIMITATION	Empowerment	*I accept the totality of who I am*	Transformation	Chi	E

EMOTION	OTHER SIDE	WAY OUT	OIL	ALARM POINT	CHART
LIMITED	Liberation	*I am willing to change*	Into the Future	Infection	B,F
LONELINESS	Connectedness with all that is	*I go to a loving space*	White Angelica	Heart	B,G,H
LONGING	Embracement	*I am receptive*	Exodus II	Heart Constrictor	C
LOSING (*Losing a battle*)	Growth	*I am aware*	Valor	Physical Body	A
LOSS	Gain	*I allow myself to give and receive*	Present Time	TMJ	B
LOSS OF SELF	*See Panic, Powerless and/or Detachment*				
LOST	Direction	*I connect with my inner knowing*	Grounding	Source	F
LOVE (*Fear of, to, or not being loveable*)	Detachment	*I allow myself to be real*	3 Wise Men	Kidney	D,G,H
LOVE (*Conditional-Agenda*)	Unconditional Love	*I view it from a higher higher perspective*	Release	Eye/Brain	B,F
MALICE	Benevolence	*I am protected*	Present Time	Heart Protector	D
MANIFESTING	Rejection	*I express*	Dream Catcher	Larynx	A,C
MANIPULATION	Understanding	*I see what is realistic*	Basil	First Rib	C,F
MASS CONSCIOUSNESS (*Being a part of*)	Manifesting Christ Consciousness	*I am conscious*	Sacred Mountain	Solar Plexus 3rd Chakra	D,G
MIND (*Overactive or Racing Mind*)	Stillness	*I allow*	Vetiver	Eye on Parietal	B
MISERABLE	Joy	*I am free*	Joy	Hepatic Duct	E
MISPERCEPTION	Understanding	*I let go of my perspective*	Acceptance	Fungus	E

EMOTION	OTHER SIDE	WAY OUT	OIL	ALARM POINT	CHART
MISS (Don't want to miss anything)	See Deprived and/or Abandonment and/or Left Behind				
MISTRUST	See Judgement				
MISUNDERSTOOD	Supported	The truth supports me	Idaho Tansy	Vocal Cords	A,B,C
MOODINESS	Stable	I am wanted and loveable	Peace & Calming	Hormone	A,E
NEGATIVE / ERRONEOUS THOUGHTS	Truth	I let go of illusions	Purification	Bacteria	D
NEGLECT, BEING NEGLECTED	See Not Good Enough				
NO PROGRESS	See Unimportant				
NOT ENOUGH	Plenty	I ask and I accept	Abundance	Heart Center	E
NOT FAIR	See Injustice				
NOT GETTING ENOUGH	Content	I am satisfied	Copaiba	Stomach	C,E,G,H
NOT GOOD ENOUGH	Acceptance	I express my best	Humility	Pericardium	E
NOT IMPORTANT	See Unimportant				
NOT MATTERING	See Unimportant				
NOT SAFE TO - Be me - Be in my body - Live in this world	Protected	I am free to: - Be me - Be in my body - Live in this world	Gratitude	Ovaries/Testes	C
NOT TRUSTING SELF	See Betrayal				
NOT WANTED	See Rejection				
NOT WANTING TO BE HERE	Being Alive	I love life	Citrus Fresh	Pancreas	C,G,H

EMOTION	OTHER SIDE	WAY OUT	OIL	ALARM POINT	CHART
NOT WORTHY	*See Worthless*				
OBLITERATION	Euphoria	*I connect my head and my heart*	Palo Santo	Throat & Heart Constrictor	A,C
OBSESSION	*See Lack*				
OBSTINATE	Motivated	*I am willing*	Mountain Savory	Liver	C,D,G,H
OPPRESSED	Free *(Finding an aspect of yourself)*	*I follow my dream*	Build Your Dream	Heart Strings	D
OUTRAGE	Regard	*I am self-sufficient*	Dill	Head of Pancreas	C,E
OVERLOADED	*See Overwhelmed*				
OVERWHELMED	Vision	*I focus my energy*	Envision	Vision	B
PAIN	Vibrant	*I am alive*	Pan Away	Injury	E,F
PANIC	Tranquility	*Peace, be still*	Trauma Life	Blood Pressure	E
PARALYZED	Motivated	*I am inspired*	Inspiration	Medulla	B,F
PARANOID	Surrender	*I am trusting*	Surrender	Esophagus	E,G
PAST *(Fear of repeating)*	Awareness	*I learn from all of life's experiences*	Forgiveness	Gallbladder	C,G,H
PATHETIC	Vibrance	*I am vibrant*	White Angelica	Aorta	C
PAYBACK	*See Revenge*				
PERSECUTED	Revered	*I express wisdom*	Valor	Kidney	D,G,H
PETRIFIED	Harmony	*I detach*	Roman Chamomile	Cervix/Penis	C

EMOTION	OTHER SIDE	WAY OUT	OIL	ALARM POINT	CHART
PHONY	Real	*I embrace life*	Cinnamon Bark	Small Intestine	E,F,G,H
PICKING UP OTHER PEOPLE'S STUFF	*See Sympathy*				
PISSED OFF	*See Anger*				
POOR	Supported	*I am expressing my passion*	Abundance	Cellular Memory	D,H
POSSESSIVENESS	Sharing	*I express*	Ylang Ylang	Laryngeal Prominence 5th Chakra	A,C
POWER *(Authority figures)*	Alignment (Spiritual)	*Spiritual conductivity*	Spikenard *or* Egyptian Gold	Nerve Root	E
POWERLESS	Powerful	*I am empowered*	Chivalry *or* Highest Potential	Kidney	D,G,H
PRIDE *(False)*	*See Injustice*				
PROCRASTINATION *(Lack of direction)*	Action	*I take action*	Lemon Myrtle	Large Intestine	D,G,H
PROTECTION *(Not having)*	Secure	*My spiritual connection protects me*	Thyme	Cellular Memory	D,H
PUNISHMENT *(Fear of, or beating self up)*	Elevated	*I accept the truth*	Harmony	Fallopian Tubes / Seminal Vesicles	C
PURPOSE *(Not fulfilling)*	Triumphance	*I am triumphant*	Vetiver	Pituitary	A,E,G,H
PUSHING *(Manifesting)*	Passion	*I express my soul*	Live with Passion	RNA	B
PUT UPON	*See Victim*				
RAGE	*See Violence*				
RAPE	*See Violence*				

EMOTION	OTHER SIDE	WAY OUT	OIL	ALARM POINT	CHART
REBELLION	Oneness	*I am one with all that is*	Release	Vertex 7th Chakra	B,C,F
RECOGNITION	Freedom	*It is safe to be seen*	Purification	Filter	B,F
REGRET / REMORSE (*Self-Blame*)	Fulfilled	*I understand this experience*	Lemon	Tonsil	B,D,H
REJECTION	Acceptance	*I accept all that I am*	Purification	Lung	C,G,H
RELENTLESS	Freedom	*I am in the flow*	Laurus Nobilis *or* White Angelica	Heart Protector	D
REPRESSED *or* STUFFED EMOTIONS	Speak Out	*I am wanted and loveable*	Present Time	Sigmoid Colon	E,G
REPRESSION	Creativity	*I change my perception*	Clarity	Ovaries/Testes	C
RESCUER	Regeneration	*I express self-reliance*	Cistus (Rose of Sharon)	Energy channel	C
RESENTMENT	Embracement	*I am wanted, loveable and I am whole*	Lemongrass	Hepatic Duct	E
RESIGNATION	Inner directed	*I am responsible*	Valor	Diaphragm	C,G
RESISTANCE (*Fear of movement*)	Openness	*I welcome change*	Surrender	Amygdala	A,C
RESOLUTION	Expansion	*I expand my awareness*	White Angelica	Transverse Fibers	B,F
RESPECT (*Lack of*)	Honor	*I allow myself to be real*	Hope	Sensory Perception	A
RESPONSIBILTY	*See Control*				
RESTRICTION	Mobility	*I am open to new experiences*	Legacy *or* Peppermint	Medulla	B,F
RETRIBUTION	*See Revenge*				

EMOTION	OTHER SIDE	WAY OUT	OIL	ALARM POINT	CHART
REVENGE	Detachment	*I forgive*	Dorado Azuil *or* Forgiveness	Pons	**A,B,D**
RIDICULE	Applauded	*I am honorable*	Orange	Heart Strings	**D**
RIGIDITY	Amusement	*It's a cosmic game*	Legacy *or* Peppermint	Heavy Metals	**E**
SABOTAGE (*By self or others*)	Re-establish	*I let go of old patterns*	Rosemary	Locus Ceruleus	**B,F**
SADNESS	Joy	*I see the humor in the situation*	Lemon	CNS/Lymph	**A,B,C**
SARCASTIC	Congruent	*I am harmonious*	Harmony	Brain	**A,B,E,G,H**
SCARCITY	Abundance	*I am in alignment with universal flow*	Abundance	Laryngeal Prominence	**A,C**
SCARED	Safe	*I am still*	Peace & Calming	Esophagus	**E,G**
SCATTERED	Centered	*I am centered*	Idaho Balsam Fir	Heart Center & Third Eye	**E**
SECRECY	*See Shame*				
SECURITY	*See Insecurity*				
SEEING (*Fear of*)	Awareness	*It is safe to see*	Purification	Eye (*on hands or feet only*)	**G,H**
SELF-BLAME	*See Regret/Remorse*				
SELF-CENTERED	Respect	*I am balanced*	Geranium	Vision	**B**
SELF-DENIAL	Wisdom	*I support myself*	Forgiveness	C1	**B,F**
SELF-DESTRUCTIVE	Valued	*I respect myself*	Melaleuca Quinquenervia	Locus Ceruleus	**B,F**
SELF-DOUBT	*See Survival and/or Powerless*				
SELF-ESTEEM (*Low*)	*See Powerless*				

EMOTION	OTHER SIDE	WAY OUT	OIL	ALARM POINT	CHART
SELF-HATRED	*See Love*				
SELF-LOATHING	*See Love*				
SELF-PITY	Secure	*I am secure*	Cardamon	Ileum	E
SELF-SACRIFICE	Understanding	*I go to the depths (core)*	ImmuPower	Cerebral Spinal Fluid	B
SEPARATE	Complete	*I am connected to _____*	Idaho Balsam Fir	Vertex 8th Chakra	B,C,F
SERVE ME	*See Entitlement*				
SETTLING SCORES	*See Revenge*				
SHAME	Understanding	*I learn from all of life's experiences*	White Angelica	Hypothalamus	A,E
SHOULD	Spontaneous	*I am guided*	Lemongrass	Tendon	B,F
SHUT DOWN	Creative	*I am vibrantly alive*	Patchouli	Brain Integration	B,F
SLAVE	*See Enslaved*				
SLUGGISH	Alive	*I allow myself to be here*	Inspiration	Bones of Ear	B
SNEAKY	Direct	*I am clear*	Thieves	Common Bile Duct	C,H
SORCERY	Ignite	*I empower*	Palo Santo	Heart Protector	D
SORROW	Peace	*I am in balance*	Acceptance	Bronchial	C,G
SPEAKING OUT (*Fear of*)	Free Will	*Not my will, but Thine*	Sacred Mountain	Throat	A
SPINNING WHEELS	*See Frustration*				
STAGNATION	Transformation	*I am empowered*	Transformation	Chi (2" Below Umbilicus)	E

EMOTION	OTHER SIDE	WAY OUT	OIL	ALARM POINT	CHART
STRESS (*Physical*)	Fun	*Life is fun*	Eucalyptus Radiata	Pleura	C
STRESS (*Emotional*)	Harmony	*I understand*	Clarity	Brain Integration	B,F
STRUGGLE	Clarity	*I accept my emotions*	Abundance	Eye on Parietal	B
STUBBORN	Flexible	*I am objective*	Chivalry or Harmony	Stomach	C,E,G,H
STUCK	Transformed	*I experience*	Lemon	Sinus	A,E,G,H
STUPID	Knowledgable	*I learn easily*	Tea Tree	Thalamus	A,B,E
SUCCESS (*Fear of*)	Acceptance	*I accept awareness*	Release	Large Intestine	D,G,H
SUFFOCATED	Breathe	*I can breathe*	Lemon	Pleura	C
SUPERIOR TO, BETTER THAN	*See Not Good Enough*				
SUPPRESSED EMOTION	*See Emotions, Suppressed*				
SUPPRESSION	Harmony	*I express my essence*	Juniper	Kidney	D,G,H
SURVIVAL	Unity	*I am one with all that is*	Cedarwood or Western Red Cedar or Canadian Red Cedar	Cervix/Penis 1st Chakra	C
SUSPICIOUS	Honest	*I am safe*	Marjoram	Raphe Nucleus	B,F
SWALLOWED EMOTIONS	*See Emotions, Swallowed*				
SWALLOWED UP	Self-Determined	*I choose my path*	Carrot Seed	Ovaries/Testes	C
SYMPATHY	Empathy	*I let go and let God/Jehovah*	White Angelica	Solar Plexus	D,G
TAKEN FOR GRANTED	Honored	*I honor myself*	Present Time	Gums/Teeth	B,E
TERROR	Safety	*I surrender*	Onycha or Sandalwood	Peritoneum	C

EMOTION	OTHER SIDE	WAY OUT	OIL	ALARM POINT	CHART
TIRED	Rejuvenated	*I am renewed*	Humility	Pancreatic Duct	E
TORMENTED	*See Victim*				
TOXICITY (*Chemical / Electro-magnetic / Emotional*)	Transformation	*Into the void*	Legacy *or* Oregano*	Connector	B
TRAPPED	Free	*I am free*	Transformation	Solar Plexus	D,G
TRAUMA	Growth	*It is safe to grow*	Relieve It	Heart Strings	D
TRUST	*See Betrayal*				
TRUTH (*Fear of hearing the*)	Listening to Spirit/God/ Jehovah/Yahweh	*I trust*	Helichrysum	Eustachian Tube	B,G
UNAPPRECIATED	Important	*I am on purpose*	JuvaFlex	Lung	C,G,H
UNCERTAIN	Focused	*I am clear and focused*	Thieves	Saliva Glands	B
UNFOLDMENT (*Fear of*)	Openness	*I allow movement*	Lavender	Raphe Nucleus	B,F
UNFULFILLED	Awareness	*I am aware of who I am*	Majoram	Posterior Fontanel	B
UNGRATEFUL	Gratitude	*I appreciate*	Ledum	Spleen	D,G,H
UNGROUNDED	Grounded	*I am stable*	Australian Blue	Bladder	C,E,G,H
UNIMPORTANT (*Being*)	Value	*I take personal responsibility*	Pine	Mucous Membrane	A,C
UNKNOWN (*Fear of the*)	Knowingness	*Listen to your heart*	Sacred Mountain	Pineal	B,F,H
UNMOTIVATED	Focused	*I am responsive*	Lime	Lung	C,G,H

---

* *Oregano can be caustic to sensitive skin, especially on the forehead. Add vegetable oil to the drop in your hand before applying to forehead, or simply touch the points on your forehead without applying oil.*

EMOTION	OTHER SIDE	WAY OUT	OIL	ALARM POINT	CHART
UNREALISTIC EXPECTATIONS	*See Expectations*				
UNRELIABILITY (Fear of life being unreliable)	Reliable	*I honor myself*	Lemon	Unconscious	B,D
UNSUPPORTED (Feeling of being)	Secure	*I take personal responsibility*	JuvaFlex or Birch or Idaho Balsam Fir or Wintergreen	Ligament	F,H
UNSURE	*See Confusion and/or Uncertain*				
UNTRUSTING	*See Judgement*				
UNWANTED	*See Rejection*				
UNWELCOME	Needed	*I am here for a purpose*	Roman Chamomile	Aorta	C
UNWORTHY (Feeling)	Worthy	*I open my heart*	Jasmine	Pons	A,B,D
USED (Being)	Respected	*I respect who I am*	Jasmine	CX@CV-5 Circulation/Sex	C,E
USELESS	Essential	*I am perfection*	Hope	Hypothalamus	A,E
VENGEANCE	*See Revenge*				
VICTIM (Consciousness)	Inner Strength (Connecting with your)	*I am cause*	Magnify Your Purpose	Allergy	C
VICTIM (Being a)	Self-responsible	*I am real*	Peace & Calming	Nerve	C,D,F
VIOLENCE	Direction	*I express peace*	Purification	Liver	C,D,G,H
VOID	*See Confusion*				

EMOTION	OTHER SIDE	WAY OUT	OIL	ALARM POINT	CHART
VULNERABLE	Whole	*I am one with all that is*	Oregano*	Reticular Activating System	B,F
WANTING TO PLEASE	Detachment	*I am loved*	Geranium	Heart Constrictor	C
WEAKNESS	Protection	*I am centered*	White Angelica	Ant. Fontanel .... B Heart Constrictor .... C Nerve .... C,D,F Filter .... B,F	
WHAT IS THE USE	*See Worthless*				
WHAT IS WRONG WITH ME	*See Not Good Enough*				
WILL (*Misuse of*)	Divinely directed	*I listen to my inner knowing*	Spikenard *or* Egyptian Gold	Disc	D
WISDOM (*Fear of*)	Illumination	*Face the fear*	Ylang Ylang	Pituitary	A,E,G,H
WISHY WASHY	Direction	*I am focused*	Citronella	Spinal Cord	B,F,H
WITHDRAWN	Detachment	*I am free*	Valor	Pineal	B,F,H
WORRY	Abundance	*I go to the depths*	Abundance	Esophagus	E,G
WORTHLESS (*Feeling*)	Approval	*I am valuable*	Frankincense	Gums/Teeth	B,E
WRONG	Knowingness	*I am true to my source*	Release	Accessory Spleen	D

---

* *Oregano can be caustic to sensitive skin, especially on the forehead. Add vegetable oil to the drop in your hand before applying to forehead, or simply touch the points on your forehead without applying oil.*

CHAKRA or ENERGY CENTERS

EMOTION	OTHER SIDE	WAY OUT	OIL	ALARM POINT	CHART

It is my intention to return my body, mind and spirit to the point of perfection.

EMOTION	OTHER SIDE	WAY OUT	OIL	ALARM POINT	CHART
SEPARATE	Complete	*I am connected to Divine Spirit/God/ Jehovah/Yahweh/ All That Is*	Idaho Balsam Fir	8" above Crown 8th Chakra	
REBELLION	Oneness	*I am one with all that is*	Release	Vertex 7th Chakra	B,C,F
CONCEIT	Meekness	*I know who I am*	Cedarwood	Hypothalamus 6th Chakra	A,E
POSSESSIVENESS	Sharing	*I express*	Ylang Ylang	Laryngeal Prominence 5th Chakra	A,C
GREED	Giving	*I am enough*	White Angelica	Ht Constrictor 4th Chakra	C
MASS CONSCIOUSNESS *(Being a part of)*	Christ Consciousness Manifesting	*I am Conscious*	Sacred Mtn.	Solar Plexus 3rd Chakra	D,G
EXPECTATIONS	Appreciating	*I am complete within myself*	SARA	Bladder 2nd Chakra	C,E,G
SURVIVAL	Unity	*I am one with all that is*	Cedarwood *or* Canadian *or* Western Red Cedar	Cervix/Penis 1st Chakra	C

Chakra or Energy Centers

Chakras are energy centers found along the mid-line of the body, extending through the torso both in the front and back. The 1st Chakra is located around the tailbone and the 7th Chakra at the top of the head, with the rest in between.

Emotions are projected and received via the energy transmitted through the chakras. Once emotions are generated or accepted into our energy field, they move through the body via the meridian system which consists of energy channels that feed all the glands, organs and systems. Emotions, like areas of the body, have specific vibrational frequencies and will accumulate in areas with the same frequency. This is why certain emotions are associated with certain areas of the body, and how the chakras are connected to the meridian system.

CHAKRA HARMONY

Toning adds an additional dimension to chakra clearing. In addition to clearing, chakras can also be balanced and the positive aspects enhanced. Toning can be used to clear depression, heal the mind and body, as well as create the life you want. Vowel sounds are used because they provide the power to the language and the musical notes set the stage.

Ideally, initially clear all the chakras on all levels by starting with the first, or root chakra, and progressing upward, ending with the eighth chakra, the base of which is located 8 inches above the top of the head.

Begin by placing a drop of the associated oil, Cedarwood, Canadian or Western Red Cedar, used for the first or root chakra, into the palm of your non-dominant hand and rotate the drop of oil clockwise three times to activate it. Next place the oil on the chakra point, in this case the pubic bone, the emotional points on the forehead, top of head, spinal cord or release point, and both filter points. Then smell the oil, feel both sides of the emotion, and say the statement or "way out." Play the note C, and tone the corresponding vowel sound "U" which is expressed as "Hu" and happens to be an ancient name for God. Breathe in a deep clearing breath and exhale, releasing any held energies. Smell the oil, feel both sides of the emotion and say the statement. Play the note and tone the vowel sound ending with a releasing, cleansing breath. Repeat a third time to clear all three layers in the front of the body.

These three layers correspond to three energy layers that extend from the physical body The first layer relates to health, or the physical energy body, it contains the energy reserves you hold for yourself. This layer is usually best felt at approximately four inches away from the body. The second layer is primarily emotional and contains the energy we have for other people. It is approximately eight inches away from the body. The 3rd layer is associated with the mental body and extends about twelve inches and beyond from the body. The three aspects of toning, sound, hearing and release, correspond to the mind, body and spirit, thus supporting and enhancing function, growth and development.

To clear all three layers in the back of the body, repeat the procedure toning C# (sharp) instead of C three times. The third, seventh and eighth chakras only have a single note (no sharp); so toning is only done three times to clear both the front and back chakras.

At the beginning of the day, clearing all the chakras with oils and toning is a great way to align your energy field or to recap and unwind before retiring for the night. The "Chakra Harmony Video" was designed to be used either actively to enhance your experience, or passively as background to soothe and balance your energy field and your environment.

For a quick pickup, test each chakra and treat only the one or ones that are out of balance. The most powerful is the eighth chakra which affects the third layer or outermost energy field and ties all the chakras and the energies they carry together. Tone three times to correct, running your hand from the top of your head down the sides, back, and front of your body, clearing your field and sealing your aura with your intention. Retest to confirm correction and determine if anything else needs to be enhanced. Enhancing the 8th chakra will balance your energy for the day, allowing you to approach the world with a clear field and attract your hearts desire. The chakras are listed on the following page with their corresponding tone and vowel sound. Both sides of the emotions and the "way out" are combined into a single statement. (You may choose to link the other emotions in a similar fashion.)

CHAKRA HARMONY TONING CHART

1st CHAKRA ROOT

Oil: Western or Canadian Red Cedar   Location: Pubic Bone   Note: Middle C, C#   Vowel Sound: Hu
I am one with all that is, which allows me to move out of **Survival** into **Unity**.

2nd CHAKRA CREATIVE

Oil: SARA   Location: Bladder   Note: D, D#   Vowel Sound: O
I am complete within myself, which allows me to release **Expectations** and move into **Appreciation**.

3rd CHAKRA SOLAR PLEXUS

Oil: Sacred Mountain   Location: Solar Plexus   Note: E   Vowel Sound: Ah
I am conscious, which allows me to move out of **Mass Consciousness** and manifest **Christ Consciousness.**

4th CHAKRA HEART

Oil: White Angelica   Location: Heart   Note: F, F#   Vowel Sound: A
I am enough, which allows me to release **Greed** and freely **Give**.

5th CHAKRA THROAT

Oil: Ylang Ylang   Location: Throat   Note: G, G#   Vowel Sound: I
I express, which allows me to release **Possessiveness** and freely **Share.**

6th CHAKRA THIRD EYE

Oil: Cedarwood   Location: Third Eye   Note: A, A#   Vowel Sound: E
I know who I am, which allows me to release **Conceit** and embody **Meekness**.

7th CHAKRA CROWN

Oil: Release   Location: Crown   Note: B   Vowel Sound: E
I am one with all that is, which allows me to release **Rebellion** and experience **Oneness.**

8th CHAKRA STAR

Oil: Idaho Balsam Fir   Location: 8" Above Crown   Note: High C   Vowel Sound: Hu
It is my intention to return my Body, Mind and Spirit to the point of Perfection.

CLEARING EMOTIONAL PATTERNS

A video demonstrating the process of releasing emotional patterns with essential oils can be found at:

www.bodytype.com/videos/videos

Changing an emotional pattern requires identifying the emotion, understanding the pattern, being aware of another way of expressing the feeling, and learning the lesson. Until we learn from an experience, we continue to recreate similar situations. Once we learn how to shift the blocked feeling, we are free.

Healing a cellular memory pattern involves awareness on all levels: mental, emotional, spiritual, and physical. Until a conditioned response is released from the body (physical/emotional) the behavior continues, like the conditioned response of Pavlov's dog. The body can be cleared by accessing the emotions through the alarm points, and the limbic system of the brain—accessed through smell.

Emotions are released by feeling both the negative and positive polarities, which allows access to both sides of the coin. Similar situations from the past will often surface; many can be released simply by acknowledging them.

The acknowledgement is brought to conscious awareness (mental/ spiritual) by identifying the emotion, its other side, and the lesson or way out of an uncomfortable state.

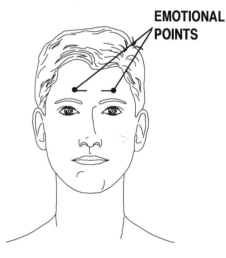

EMOTIONAL POINTS

Clearing Procedure
1. identify and **FEEL** the EMOTION,

2. smell the appropriate OIL, taking it into all your cells,

3. **FEEL** the OTHER SIDE of the emotion,

4. apply the oil to the ALARM POINT(S),

5. apply the oil to or simply touch the EMOTIONAL POINTS on the frontal eminences,

6. focus on or say the STATEMENT that provides a way out, this allows you to move from a negative to a positive state, continue breathing the oil until you feel the energy shift,

7. repeat as needed, may be once, 3, 7, 10 or 18 times (which is essentially every waking hour) for 1, 3, or 7 weeks, essentially until the pattern is no longer present in your life.

Note: Application frequency is determined by the depth of the emotional pattern. The quickest way to clear deep seated or core issues is 18 times per day for 7 weeks, but remember, you are free to choose your pace. The length of time is immaterial. Whether you take 7 weeks or 7 months is up to you. Since every waking hour is often impractical, the procedure can be done as close as every 15 minutes allowing you to do it perhaps 4 to 6 times before work, several times during the day and complete it at night when you get home.

Doing the clearing procedure at night before you go to bed allows your subconscious to process the emotional patterns during your dream state. By applying the oil or oils to a diffuser by your bed or on a cotton ball on your pillow allows you to continue to breathe the oil while you sleep. Additional ways to reduce application frequency are to include the oils in your bath or shower, and before meditation or exercise.

Since some of the alarm points on the body are hard to access, such as the liver point, you may wish to use the corresponding point on the hands at times. Refer to the hand chart for the exact location.

As emotions surface, they need to be released. Writing, talking, exercise, salt or sweat baths are helpful. If the emotional release becomes too intense, reduce the frequency or take a break and extend time. Corresponding or related emotions may need to be addressed before a core issue can be completely cleared.

You can treat different emotions that use the same oil or related emotions that use different oils. One oil and/or emotion can immediately follow another. Clear all the emotions as they surface, treat until emotional charge is gone and the pattern is released. Honor yourself and pay attention to what is best you.

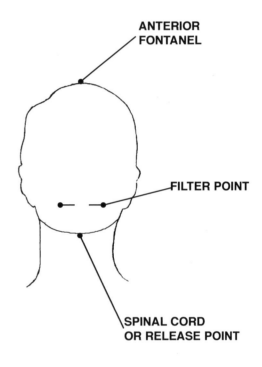

Oil Sensitivity
Some oils are strong and may be irritating to sensitive skin, especially on the face and forehead. If you experience drying or burning, dilute the oil using V6 or any vegetable oil. If you experience any difficulty with the oils, simply smell the oil and touch the alarm and emotional points, feeling the emotions and saying the statement.

Certain oils like *Lemon* can cause a person to be photosensitive, burning easily in bright sunlight. Use these oils with caution, smelling rather than applying.

Once the oil has been used, feeling the feelings and saying the statement is often effective when using the oil is inconvenient.

The most important element is your intention. Feel the feelings and focus on the statement. There may be times when the statement is unclear. As you work with it, a new awareness will surface. This is a learning, unfolding process.

Enhancement to Clearing Procedure
Once the essential oil has been applied to the alarm points and the frontal eminences, it can also be applied to the Anterior Fontanel, Spinal Cord or Release point at the base of the skull, and to the Filter points on both sides of the back of the skull.

The Release point assists in releasing the emotional pattern, and the Filter points serve to filter energies that would pull a person back into the old pattern.

VARIATION OF CLEARING EMOTIONAL PATTERNS[10]
(WITHOUT MUSCLE TESTING)

1. Feel the emotion. Totally embody it. (If you are highly emotional and concerned about getting "stuck" in the emotion, afraid you will not be able to get out of it, be reassured that this technique will help clear the emotion.)

2. Take a deep breath and inhale the appropriate oil, repeat three (3) times.

3. Feel the other side of the emotion.

4. Apply the oil to the alarm point(s).

5. Apply the oil to the emotional points on the frontal eminences, the spinal cord or release point, the filter points on the back of the head, and the anterior fontanel on the top of the head.

6. Say the statement out loud, repeating it until you feel the energy blocks release and you come to a point of stillness.

7. Then mouth the statement, without making any sound. (Actually make the movements with your mouth, but without making sound. This does not work if you just mentally say it in your head.) Repeat mouthing the statement until the energy blocks release and you again come to a point of stillness[10].

8. Finish by mentally saying the statement to yourself three (3) times.

9. Repeat this procedure whenever this or any other negative emotion surfaces, or an emotional energy block emerges.

CLEARING PROCEDURE FOR CHILDREN

Procedure to Clear Anger in Children
Hold the oil under the child's nose, allowing the child to smell it. In the case of Anger, the oil is *Purification*. Acknowledge the emotion by saying, "You're feeling angry, aren't you?" "Yeah" or no response. Put a drop of *Purification* in the palm of your non-dominant hand and rotate the drop 3 times clockwise to activate the oil. Touch the liver alarm point on both the left and right hands and say, "The other side of anger is laughter," and smile.

Touch the two emotional points on the forehead with *Purification* oil on your fingers or place the palm of your hand (with the oil) on the child's forehead over the emotional points and say, "The way to move from anger to laughter is 'My direction is clear'." If appropriate you may ask the child to say, "My direction is clear."

Repeat the procedure as often as appropriate. It is beneficial to treat yourself immediately before or after treating the child (includes adult children), as it helps build the child's sense of self-esteem. By including yourself, the child is not made to feel that something is "wrong" with him or her, but that emotions are part of life and we can choose how we express our feelings.

---

[10] Contributed by Susan Ulfelder, N.D.

Oils Reference

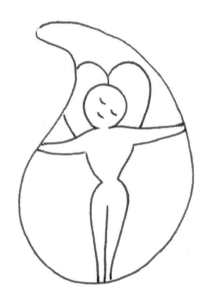

OILS REFERENCE
OILS, EMOTIONS AND BODY ALARM POINTS

OIL	EMOTION	ALARM POINT
ABUNDANCE	Not Enough	Heart Center
ABUNDANCE	Poor	Cellular Memory
ABUNDANCE	Scarcity	Laryngeal Prominence
ABUNDANCE	Struggle	Eye on Parietal
ABUNDANCE	Worry	Esophagus
ACCEPTANCE	Don't Belong	Solar Plexus
ACCEPTANCE	Embarrassed	Hypothalamus
ACCEPTANCE	Insecurity	Ileum
ACCEPTANCE	Misperception	Fungus
ACCEPTANCE	Sorrow	Bronchial
AROMA LIFE	Aloneness	Heart Protector
AROMA SIEZ	Inconsistency	Unconscious
AUSTRALIAN BLUE	Disgust	Bronchial
AUSTRALIAN BLUE	Ungrounded	Bladder
AWAKEN	Connecting Interdimensionally	Sacral Door
AWAKEN	Expansion	Soul Integration
AWAKEN	Hopelessness	Bone Marrow
BASIL	Manipulation	First Rib
BELIEVE	Dishonesty	Spleen
BLUE TANSY *or* IDAHO TANSY	Intimidated	Hormone
BRAIN POWER *or* GENEYUS	Apathy	Hippocampus
BRAIN POWER *or* GENEYUS	Brain Fog	Brain *or* Roof of Mouth
BUILD YOUR DREAM	Oppressed	Heart Strings
CANADIAN *or* WESTERN RED CEDAR	Incompletion	Will @ C-5
CANADIAN *or* WESTERN RED CEDAR *or* CEDARWOOD	Survival	Cervix/Penis – 1st Chakra
CARDAMON	Self-Pity	Ileum
CARROT SEED	Swallowed Up	Ovaries/Testes

OIL	EMOTION	ALARM POINT
CASSIA	Dependent	Will @ C5
CEDARWOOD	Conceit	Hypothalamus – 6th Chakra
CELERY SEED	Ambivalence	Hippocampus
CHIVALRY or HIGHEST POTENTIAL	Powerless	Kidney
CHIVALRY or HARMONY	Stubborn	Stomach
CINNAMON BARK	Irritation	Head of Pancreas
CINNAMON BARK	Phony	Small Intestine
CISTUS (ROSE OF SHARON)	Rescuer	Energy Channel
CITRONELLA	Wishy Washy	Spinal Cord
CITRUS FRESH	Not Wanting to be Here	Pancreas
CLARITY	Emotional Stress	Brain Integration
CLARITY	Guilt	Spleen
CLARITY	Repression	Ovaries Testes
CLARY SAGE	Intolerance, General	Toxic
CLOVE	Lashing Out	Tongue
COMMON SENSE	Controlling by Attacking	Ileum
COPAIBA	Lies	Spinal Cord
COPAIBA	Not Getting Enough	Stomach
CYPRESS	Disrespect	Veins
DI-GIZE or DI-TONE	Disillusioned	Appendix
DILL	Outrage	Head of Pancreas
DORADO AZUIL	Revenge	Pons
DREAM CATCHER	Competitiveness	Lymph Valves
DREAM CATCHER	Fear of Manifesting	Larynx
EGYPTIAN GOLD or SPIKENARD	Power (Authority figure)	Nerve Root
EGYPTIAN GOLD or SPIKENARD	Will (Misuse of)	Disc
ELEMI	Diabolical Disorientation	3rd Eye
ENDOFLEX	Denial	Vision

OIL	EMOTION	ALARM POINT
EN-R-GEE	Isolation	Yeast/Umbilicus
ENVISION	Attachment	Vision
ENVISION	Confined	Intuative
ENVISION	Overwhelmed	Vision
EUCALYPTUS BLUE	Frozen	Bladder
EUCALYPTUS BLUE	Suppressed Emotion	Eye/Brain on Occipit
EUCALYPTUS (GLOBULUS)	Bondage	Parotid
EUCALYPTUS (RADIATA)	Physical Stress	Pleura
EXODUS II	Complaisance	Magic
EXODUS II	Doomed	Solar Plexus
EXODUS II	Longing	Heart Constrictor
FORGIVENESS	Betrayal	Pancreas
FORGIVENESS	Distrust	Uterus/Prostate
FORGIVENESS	Repeating the Past	Gallbladder
FORGIVENESS	Revenge	Pons
FORGIVENESS	Self-Denial	CI
FRANKINCENSE	Dizziness *(Vertigo)*	Ear, Middle
FRANKINCENSE	Feelings of Worthlessness	Gums/Teeth
FRANKINCENSE	"F- YOU"	Ego
GATHERING	Bad *(Feeling)*	Kidney
GATHERING	Enslaved	Meninges
GENEYUS *or* BRAIN POWER	Apathy	Hippocampus
GENEYUS *or* BRAIN POWER	Brain Fog	Brain or Roof of Mouth
GERANIUM	Self-Centered	Vision
GERANIUM	Wanting to Please	Heart Constrictor
GERMAN CHAMOMILE	Disassociation	Soul (C2)
GINGER	Lack	Peyer's Patches
GOLDENROD	Defenseless	Adrenal Cortex
GRAPEFRUIT	Distress	Heart Strings
GRATITUDE	Not Safe to *(Be me, Be in my body, Live in this world)*	Ovaries/Testes

OIL	EMOTION	ALARM POINT
GROUNDING	Boredom	Parasites
GROUNDING	Lost	Source
HARMONY	Being Ignored	Strep
HARMONY	Crushed	Blood
HARMONY	Hostility	Harmony
HARMONY	Punishment *(Fear of)*/ Beating Self Up	Fallopian Tubes/ Seminal Vesicles
HARMONY	Sarcastic	Brain
HARMONY or CHIVALRY	Stubborn	Stomach
HELICHRYSUM	Fear of Death/Living	Arteries
HELICHRYSUM	Fear of Hearing the Truth	Eustachian Tube
HELICHRYSUM	Integrity *(Lack of)*	Brain
HELICHRYSUM	Irresponsible	Eustachian Tube
HIGHEST POTENTIAL	Annoyance	Courage
HIGHEST POTENTIAL	Get Even	Thyroid
HIGHEST POTENTIAL or CHIVALRY	Powerless	Kidney
HINOKI	Incapacitated	Bone-Center of Sacrum
HOPE	Blindness	Eye Lymph
HOPE	Lack of Respect	Sensory Perception
HOPE	Useless	Hypothalamus
HUMILITY	Being, Less than	Medulla
HUMILITY	Not good enough	Pericardium
HUMILITY	Tired	Pancreatic Duct
HYSSOP	Swallowed Emotions	Epiglottis
IDAHO BALSAM FIR	Inadequate	GV-20
IDAHO BALSAM FIR	Scattered	Heart Center & Third Eye
IDAHO BALSAM FIR	Separate	Vertex – 8th Chakra
IDAHO BALSAM FIR	Unsupported	Ligament
IMMUPOWER	Self -Sacrifice	Cerebral Spinal Fluid
INNER CHILD	Clearing Cellular Memory	DNA

OIL	EMOTION	ALARM POINT
INNER CHILD	Desertion	RNA
INNER CHILD	Distortion	Innocence
INNER CHILD	Erratic Energy	Duodenum
INSPIRATION	Fatigue	Life Force
INSPIRATION	Paralyzed	Medulla
INSPIRATION	Sluggish	Ear, Bones of
INTO THE FUTURE	Limited	Infection
JASMINE	Being Used	CX @ CV-5
JASMINE	Feeling Unworthy	Pons
JOY	Anxiety	Capillary
JOY	Disappointment	Bronchial
JOY	Grief	Adenoids
JOY	Incongruency	Ears, External
JOY	Judgment	Solar Plexus
JOY	Miserable	Hepatic Duct
JUNIPER	Suppression	Kidney
JUVA FLEX	Blame	Toxic
JUVA FLEX	Unappreciated	Lung
JUVAFLEX *or* BIRCH	Deprived	Joints/Cartilage
JUVAFLEX *or* BIRCH	Feeling of Being Unsupported	Ligament
JUVAFLEX *or* BIRCH	Rebelling Against *or* Resentment of Authority	Bone
LAURUS NOBILIS *or* WHITE ANGELICA	Consciousness Shifting	Aorta
LAURUS NOBILIS *or* WHITE ANGELICA	Relentless	Heart Protector
LAVENDER	Abandonment	Small Intestine
LAVENDER	Criticism	Skin
LAVENDER	Fear of Unfoldment	Raphe Nucleus
LEGACY *or* MYRRH	Difficulty	PSIS
LEGACY *or* PEPPERMINT	Rigidity	Heavy Metals

OIL	EMOTION	ALARM POINT
LEGACY *or* OREGANO	Toxicity *(Chemical, Electromagnetic, Emotional)*	Connector
LEDUM	Dissatisfaction	Magic
LEDUM	Hate *or* Hatred	Hepatic Duct
LEDUM	Ungrateful	Spleen
LEMON	Being Left Behind	Lymph
LEMON	Entitlement	Parathyroid
LEMON	Fear of Detachment	Spinal Cord
LEMON	Feeling of Emptiness	Breast
LEMON	Frustration	Common Bile Duct
LEMON	Life Being Unreliable	Unconscious
LEMON	Regret/Remorse	Tonsil
LEMON	Sadness	CNS/Lymph
LEMON	Stuck	Sinus
LEMON	Suffocated	Pleura
LEMONGRASS	Resentment	Hepatic Duct
LEMONGRASS	Should	Tendon
LEMON MYRTLE	Procrastination	Large Intestine
LIME	Belittled	Vision
LIME	Unmotivated	Lung
LIVE WITH PASSION	Dread	Arteries
LIVE WITH PASSION	Hurt	Creativity
LIVE WITH PASSION	Pushing	RNA
LONGEVITY	Choked	Vibration
MAGNIFY YOUR PURPOSE	Confusion	Integration
MAGNIFY YOUR PURPOSE	Confusion	Integration
MAGNIFY YOUR PURPOSE	Victim Consciousness	Allergy
MARJORAM	Disconnected	Umbilicus/Yeast
MARJORAM	Suspicious	Raphe Nucleus
MARJORAM	Unfulfilled	Posterior Fontanel

OIL	EMOTION	ALARM POINT
MELALEUCA ERICIFOLIA (ROSALINA) *or* TEA TREE	Disempowered	C1
MELALEUCA QUINQUENERVIA	Self-Destructive	Locus Ceruleus
MELROSE	Impatience	Immune
MELROSE	Injury	Periosteum
MOTIVATION	Inertia	Courage
MOUNTAIN SAVORY	Obstinate	Liver
MYRRH	Fear of Facing the World	Adrenal
MYRRH *or* LEGACY	Difficulty	PSIS
MYRTLE	Suppression of Life	Chi
NUTMEG *or* EN-R-GEE	Adrenal Exhaustion	Adrenal
OCOTEA	Insulted	Ego
ONYCHA *or* SANDALWOOD	Terror	Peritoneum
ORANGE	Ridicule	Heart Strings
OREGANO	Fear of Completion	Anterior Fontanel
OREGANO *or* LEGACY	Toxicity	Connector
OREGANO	Vunerable	Reticluar Activating System
PALO SANTO	Anguish	Heart
PALO SANTO	Limbo	3rd Eye
PALO SANTO	Obliteration	Throat & Heart Constrictor
PALO SANTO	Sorcery	Heart Protector
PANAWAY	Exhaustion	Muscle
PANAWAY	Fear of Emotions	Fascia
PANAWAY	Pain	Injury
PATCHOULI	Shut Down	Brain Integration
PEACE & CALMING (II)	Addiction	Brain
PEACE & CALMING (II)	Argumentiveness	Thyroid
PEACE & CALMING (II)	Being a Victim	Nerve
PEACE & CALMING (II)	Depression	Depression
PEACE & CALMING (II)	Indecisiveness	Higher Will @ C-3

OIL	EMOTION	ALARM POINT
PEACE & CALMING (II)	Control	Stomach
PEACE & CALMING (II)	Moodiness	Hormone
PEACE & CALMING (II)	Scared	Esophagus
PEPPER, BLACK	Being in a Black Hole	Temporal Bone, Mastoid Portion
PEPPERMINT	Failure	Thymus
PEPPERMINT	Fear of Dependence	Thalamus
PEPPERMINT	Restriction	Medulla
PEPPERMINT *or* LEGACY	Rigidity	Heavy Metals (ASIS)
PINE	Being Unimportant	Mucous Membranes
PINE	Degraded	White Blood Cells
PRESENT TIME	Flustered	Periosteum
PRESENT TIME	Illusion	Virus
PRESENT TIME	Loss	TMJ
PRESENT TIME	Malice	Heart Protector
PRESENT TIME	Repressed *or* Stuffed Emotions	Sigmoid Colon
PRESENT TIME	Resistance to Change	Rectum
PRESENT TIME	Taken for Granted	Gums/Teeth
PURIFICATION	Anger	Liver
PURIFICATION	Being Alone	Staph
PURIFICATION	Fear of Rejection	Lung
PURIFICATION	Fear of Seeing	Eye *(On hands and feet only)*
PURIFICATION	Negative *or* Erroneous Thoughts	Bacteria
PURIFICATION	Recognition	Filter
PURIFICATION	Violence	Liver
RAVENSARA	Deceived	Eye/Brain on Occipit
RC	Depletion	Lymphatic Congestion
RELEASE	Dejection	Pleura
RELEASE	Fear of Success	Large Intestine
RELEASE	Holding Back *(Universal flow)*	Trachea
RELEASE	Loss of Identity	Uterus/Prostate

OIL	EMOTION	ALARM POINT
RELEASE	Love Being Conditional – Agenda	Eye/Brain on Occiput
RELEASE	Rebellion	Vertex – 7th Chakra
RELEASE	Wrong	Accessory Spleen
RELIEVE IT	Trauma	Heart Strings
ROMAN CHAMOMILE	Petrified	Cervix/Penis
ROMAN CHAMOMILE	Unwelcome	Aorta
ROSE	Disintegrated	Virus
ROSE	Fear of Intimacy	Heart Center
ROSEMARY	Sabotage, By Self *or* Others	Locus Ceruleus
ROSEWOOD	Agitated	Blood Pressure
ROSEWOOD	Blindsided	Temporal Bone, Mastoid Portion
RUTAVALA	Frightened	Ego
RUTAVALA	Lifeless	Hara
SACRED MOUNTAIN	Being a part of Mass Consciousness	Solar Plexus – 3rd Chakra
SACRED MOUNTAIN	Compromising Self	Soul
SACRED MOUNTAIN	Fear of Hearing	Ears, Inner
SACRED MOUNTAIN	Fear of Speaking Out	Throat
SACRED MOUNTAIN	Fear of the Unknown	Pineal
SACRED MOUNTAIN	Injustice	Thyroid
SAGE	Letting Go	Bladder
SANDALWOOD	Co-Dependency	Emotional Integration
SANDALWOOD	Dread	Arteries
SANDALWOOD	Faith (*Lack of*)	3rd Eye
SANDALWOOD	Fear	3rd Eye
SANDALWOOD	Terror	Peritoneum
SARA	Abuse	Cellular Memory
SARA	Acceptance	Emotional point
SARA	Expectations	Bladder 2nd Chakra
SPEARMINT	Lazy	Pancreatic Duct

OIL	EMOTION	ALARM POINT
SPIKENARD *or* MELISSA	Estranged	Heart Strings
SPIKENARD *or* EGYPTIAN GOLD	Will *(Misuse of)*	Disc
SPIKENARD *or* EGYPTIAN GOLD	Power *(Authority figures)*	Nerve Root
SURRENDER	Paranoid	Esophagus
SURRENDER	Resistance *(Fear of movement)*	Amygdala
TEA TREE *or* MELALEUCA ERICIFOLIA (ROSALINA)	Disempowered	C1
TEA TREE *or* MELALEUCA ERICIFOLIA (ROSALINA)	Stupid	Thalamus
3 WISE MEN	Despair	Diaphragm
3 WISE MEN	Fear of Love *(Fear to,* or *Fear of not being loveable)*	Kidney
3 WISE MEN	Inferiority	ICV- Ileocecal Valve
TANSY, IDAHO	Misunderstood	Vocal Cords
THIEVES	Different	Mold
THIEVES	Sneaky	Common Bile Duct
THIEVES	Uncertain	Saliva Glands
THYME	No Protection	Cellular Memory
TRANSFORMATION	Can't	Virus
TRANSFORMATION	Commitment	Ego
TRANSFORMATION	Cynicism	Small Intestine
TRANSFORMATION	Limitation	Chi
TRANSFORMATION	Stagnation	Chi
TRANSFORMATION	Trapped	Solar Plexus
TRAUMA LIFE	Panic	Blood Pressure
TSUGA	Defeated	CNS/Lymph
VALOR (II)	Aggression	Adrenal Cortex
VALOR (II)	Defensiveness	Stomach

OIL	EMOTION	ALARM POINT
VALOR (II)	Fear of Conflict	Adrenal Cortex
VALOR (II)	Inability to Cope	White Blood Cells
VALOR (II)	Losing a Battle	Physical Body
VALOR (II)	Persecuted	Kidney
VALOR (II)	Resignation	Diaphragm
VALOR (II)	Withdrawn	Pineal
VETIVER	Mind, Overactive *or* Racing Mind	Eye on Parietal
VETIVER	Purpose *(Not fulfilling)*	Pituitary
WESTERN *or* CANADIAN RED CEDAR *or* CEDARWOOD	Incompletion	Will @ C-5
WESTERN *or* CANADIAN RED CEDAR *or* CEDARWOOD	Survival	Cervix/Penis – 1st Chakra
WHITE ANGELICA *or* LAURUS NOBILIS	Consciousness Shifting	Aorta
WHITE ANGELICA	Crisis	Esophagus
WHITE ANGELICA	Disharmony	Parathyroid
WHITE ANGELICA	Greed	Heart Constrictor – 4th Chakra
WHITE ANGELICA	Loneliness	Heart
WHITE ANGELICA	Pathetic	Aorta
WHITE ANGELICA *or* LAURUS NOBILIS	Rejection	Lung
WHITE ANGELICA *or* LAURUS NOBILIS	Relentless	Heart Protector
WHITE ANGELICA	Resolution	Transverse Fibers
WHITE ANGELICA	Shame	Hypothalamus
WHITE ANGELICA	Sympathy	Solar Plexus
WHITE ANGELICA	Weakness	Anterior Fontanel, Heart Constrictor, Nerve, Filter
WHITE FIR	Inadequate	GV-20
WINTERGREEN	Unsupported	Ligament
YLANG YLANG	Drained	Heart Strings

OIL	EMOTION	ALARM POINT
YLANG YLANG	Fear of Wisdom	Pituitary
YLANG YLANG	Possessiveness	Laryngeal Prominence – 5thChakra

Body Reference

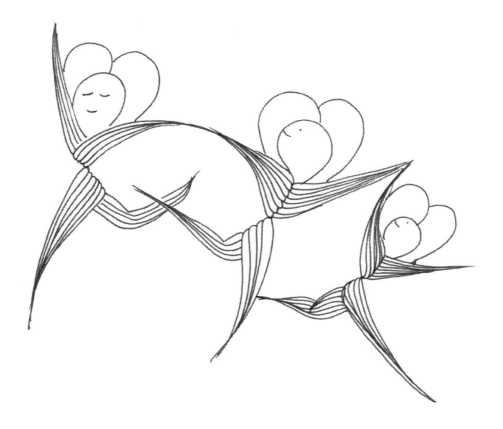

BODY REFERENCE
Body Alarm Points with Emotions and Related Oils

ALARM POINT	OIL	EMOTION
ACCESSORY SPLEEN	Release	Wrong
ADENOIDS	Joy	Grief
ADRENAL	Myrrh	Fear of Facing the World
ADRENAL	Nutmeg *or* En-R-Gee	Adrenal Exhaustion
ADRENAL CORTEX	Goldenrod	Defenseless
ADRENAL CORTEX	Valor	Aggression
ADRENAL CORTEX	Valor	Fear of Conflict
ALLERGY	Magnify Your Purpose	Victim Consciousness
AMYGDALA	Surrender	Resistance *(Fear of Movement)*
ANTERIOR FONTANEL	Oregano	Fear of Completion
ANTERIOR FONTANEL	Patchouli	Defiance
ANTERIOR FONTANEL	White Angelica	Weakness
AORTA	Lauris Nobilis *or* White Angelica	Consciousness Shifting
AORTA	Roman Chamomile	Unwelcome
AORTA	Lauris Nobilis *or* White Angelica	Pathetic
APPENDIX	Di-Gize *or* Di-Tone	Disillusioned
ARTERIES	Helichrysum	Fear of Death *(Living)*
ARTERIES	Live with Passion *or* Sandalwood	Dread
BACTERIA	Purification	Negative *or* Erroneous Thoughts
BLADDER	Australian Blue	Ungrounded
BLADDER	Eucalyptus Blue	Frozen
BLADDER	Sage	Letting Go
BLADDER – 2nd Chakra	SARA	Expectations
BLOOD	Harmony	Crushed
BLOOD PRESSURE	Rosewood	Agitated
BLOOD PRESSURE	Trauma Life	Panic

ALARM POINT	OIL	EMOTION
BONE	Birch *or* Juva Flex	Rebelling Against *or* Resentment of Authority
BONE-CENTER OF SACRUM	Hinoki	Incapacitated
BONE MARROW	Awaken	Hopelessness
BONES OF EAR	Inspiration	Sluggish
BRAIN	Harmony	Sarcastic
BRAIN	Helichrysm	Integrity *(Lack of)*
BRAIN	Peace & Calming	Addiction
BRAIN INTEGRATION	Clarity	Emotional Stress
BRAIN INTEGRATION	Patchouli	Shut Down
BREAST	Lemon	Feeling of Emptiness
BRONCHIAL	Acceptance	Sorrow
BRONCHIAL	Australian Blue	Disgust
BRONCHIAL	Joy	Disappointment
CI	Forgiveness	Self-Denial
CI	Melaleuca Ericifolia (Rosalina) *or* Tea Tree	Disempowered
CAPILLARY	Joy	Anxiety
CELLULAR MEMORY	Abundance	Poor
CELLULAR MEMORY	SARA	Abuse *(All/Any; Sexual, Ritual, Emotional)*
CELLULAR MEMORY	Thyme	No Protection
CEREBRAL SPINAL FLUID	ImmuPower	Self - Sacrifice
CERVIX/PENIS – 1st Chakra	Cedarwood *or* Western *or* Canadian Red Cedar	Survival
CERVIX/PENIS	Roman Chamomile	Petrified
CHI	Myrtle	Suppression of life
CHI	Transformation	Limitation
CHI	Transformation	Stagnation
CNS/LYMPH	Lemon	Sadness
CNS/LYMPH	Tsuga	Defeated
COMMON BILE DUCT	Lemon	Frustration

ALARM POINT	OIL	EMOTION
COMMON BILE DUCT	Thieves	Sneaky
CONNECTOR	Legacy *or* Oregano	Toxicity *(Chemical, Electromagnetic, Emotional)*
COURAGE	Highest Potential	Annoyance
COURAGE	Motivation	Inertia
CREATIVITY	Live With Passion	Hurt
CX @ CV-5	Jasmine	Being Used
DEPRESSION	Peace & Calming	Depression
DIAPHRAGM	3 Wise Men	Despair
DIAPHRAGM	Valor	Resignation
DISC	Spikenard	Misuse of Will
DNA	Inner Child	Clearing Cellular Memory
DUODENUM	Inner Child	Erratic Energy
EAR, BONES OF	Inspiration	Sluggish
EAR, EXTERNAL	Joy	Fear of Incongruency
EAR, INNER	Sacred Mountain	Fear of Hearing
EAR, MIDDLE	Frankincense	Dizziness *(Vertigo)*
EGO	Frankincense	"F-You"
EGO	Ocotea	Insulted
EGO	RutaVaLa	Frightened
EGO	Transformation	Commitment
EMOTIONAL INTEGRATION	Sandalwood	Co-Dependency
EMOTIONAL POINT	SARA	Acceptance
ENERGY CHANNEL	Cistus (Rose of Sharon)	Rescuer
EPIGLOTTIS	Hyssop	Swallowed Emotions
ESOPHAGUS	Abundance	Worry
ESOPHAGUS	Peace & Calming	Scared
ESOPHAGUS	Surrender	Paranoid
ESOPHAGUS	White Angelica	Crisis
EUSTACHIAN TUBE	Helichrysum	Fear of Hearing the Truth
EUSTACHIAN TUBE	Helichrysum	Irresponsible

ALARM POINT	OIL	EMOTION
EYE, 3rd	Sandalwood	Faith *(Lack of)*
EYE *(On hands* or *feet only)*	Purification	Fear of Seeing
EYE/BRAIN on OCCIPIT	Eucalyptus Blue	Suppressed Emotion
EYE/BRAIN on OCCIPIT	Ravensara	Deceived
EYE/BRAIN on OCCIPIT	Release	Agenda — Love being conditional
EYE on PARIETAL	Abundance	Struggle
EYE on PARIETAL	Vetiver	Mind, Overactive *or* Racing Mind
EYE LYMPH	Hope	Blindness
FALLOPIAN TUBES/ SEMINAL VESICLES	Harmony	Fear of Punishment *or* Beating Self Up
FASCIA	PanAway	Fear of Emotions
FILTER	Purification	Recognition
FILTER	White Angelica	Weakness
FIRST RIB	Basil	Manipulation
FUNGUS	Acceptance	Misperception
GALLBLADDER	Forgiveness	Fear of Repeating the Past
GUMS/TEETH	Frankincense	Feelings of Being Worthless
GUMS/TEETH	Present Time	Taken for Granted
GV-20	White Fir *or* Idaho Balsam Fir	Inadequate
HARA	RutaVaLa	Lifeless
HARMONY	Harmony	Hostility
HARMONY	White Lotus	Harmony
HEAD OF PANCREAS	Cinnamon Bark	Irritation
HEAD OF PANCREAS	Dill	Outrage
HEART	Palo Santo	Anguish
HEART	White Angelica	Loneliness
HEART CENTER	Abundance	Not Enough
HEART CENTER	Rose	Fear of Intimacy
HEART CENTER & THIRD EYE	Idaho Balsam Fir	Scattered
HEART CONSTRICTOR	Exodus II	Longing
HEART CONSTRICTOR	Geranium	Wanting to Please

ALARM POINT	OIL	EMOTION
HEART CONSTRICTOR	Palo Santo	Obliteration
HEART CONSTRICTOR	White Angelica	Weakness
HEART CONSTRICTOR – 4th Chakra	White Angelica	Greed
HEART PROTECTOR	Aroma Life	Aloneness
HEART PROTECTOR	Laurus Nobilis or White Angelica	Relentless
HEART PROTECTOR	Palo Santo	Sorcery
HEART PROTECTOR	Present Time	Malice
HEART STRINGS	Build Your Dream	Oppressed
HEART STRINGS	Grapefruit	Distress
HEART STRINGS	Orange	Ridicule
HEART STRINGS	Relieve It	Trauma
HEART STRINGS	Spikenard or Melissa	Estranged
HEART STRINGS	Ylang Ylang	Drained
HEAVY METALS	Legacy or Peppermint	Rigidity
HEPATIC DUCT	Joy	Miserable
HEPATIC DUCT	Ledum	Hate or Hatred
HEPATIC DUCT	Lemongrass	Resentment
HIGHER WILL @ C-3	Peace & Calming	Indecisiveness
HIPPOCAMPUS	Brain Power or GeneYus	Apathy
HIPPOCAMPUS	Celery Seed	Ambivalence
HORMONE	Blue Tansy or Idaho Tansy	Intimidated
HORMONE	Peace & Calming	Moodiness
HYPOTHALAMUS	Acceptance	Embarrassed
HYPOTHALAMUS – 6th Chakra	Cedarwood	Conceit
HYPOTHALAMUS	Hope	Useless
HYPOTHALAMUS	White Angelica	Fear of Shame
ICV-ILEOCECAL VALVE	3 Wise Men	Fear of Inferiority
ILEUM	Acceptance	Insecurity
ILEUM	Cardamon	Self-Pity

ALARM POINT	OIL	EMOTION
ILEUM	Common Sense	Controlling by Attacking
IMMUNE	Melrose	Impatience
INFECTION	Into the Future	Limited
INJURY	PanAway	Pain
INNER EAR	Sacred Mountain	Fear of Hearing
INNOCENCE	Cistus *(Rose of Sharon)*	Rescuer
INNOCENCE	Inner Child	Distortion
INTEGRATION	Magnify Your Purpose	Confusion
INTUITIVE	Envision	Confined
JOINTS/CARTILAGE	JuvaFlex *or* Birch	Deprived
KIDNEY	Chivalry *or* Highest Potential	Powerless
KIDNEY	Gathering	Bad *(Feeling)*
KIDNEY	Juniper	Suppression
KIDNEY	Valor	Persecuted
KIDNEY	3 Wise Men	Fear of Love *(Fear to love, Fear of loving, or Not being loveable)*
LARGE INTESTINE	Lemon Myrtle	Procrastination
LARGE INTESTINE	Release	Fear of Success
LARYNGEAL PROMINENCE	Abundance	Scarcity
LARYNGEAL PROMINENCE – 5th Chakra	Ylang Ylang	Possessiveness
LARYNX	Dream Catcher	Fear of Manifesting
LIFE FORCE	Inspiration	Fatigue
LIGAMENT	Birch *or* JuvaFlex *or* Idaho Balsam Fir *or* Wintergreen	Feeling Unsupported
LIVER	Mountain Savory	Obstinate
LIVER	Purification	Anger
LIVER	Purification	Violence
LOCUS CERULEUS	Melaleuca Quinquenervia	Self-Destructive
LOCUS CERULEUS	Rosemary	Sabotage *(By self* or *others)*

ALARM POINT	OIL	EMOTION
LUNG	JuvaFlex	Unappreciated
LUNG	Lime	Unmotivated
LUNG	Purification	Rejection
LYMPH	Lemon	Being Left Behind
LYMPHATIC CONGESTION	RC	Depletion
LYMPH VALVES	Dream Catcher	Competitiveness
MAGIC	Exodus II	Complaisance
MAGIC	Ledum	Dissatisfaction
MEDULLA	Humility	Being Less Than
MEDULLA	Inspiration	Paralyzed
MEDULLA	Peppermint	Restriction
MENINGES	Gathering	Enslaved
MIDDLE EAR	Frankincense	Dizziness (Vertigo)
MOLD	Thieves	Different
MUCOUS MEMBRANES	Pine	Being Unimportant
MUSCLE	PanAway	Exhaustion
NERVE	Peace & Calming	Being a Victim
NERVE	White Angelica	Weakness
NERVE ROOT	Spikenard	Power (Authority Figures)
OVARIES/TESTES	Carrot Seed	Swallowed Up
OVARIES/TESTES	Clarity	Repression
OVARIES/TESTES	Gratitude	Not Safe to (Be me, Be in my body, or Live in this world)
PANCREAS	Citrus Fresh	Not Wanting to be Here
PANCREAS	Forgiveness	Betrayal
PANCREATIC DUCT	Humility	Tired
PANCREATIC DUCT	Spearmint	Lazy
PARASITES	Gounding	Boredom
PARATHYROID	Lemon	Entitlement
PARATHYROID	White Angelica	Disharmony
PAROTID	Eucalyptus, Globulus	Fear of Bondage

ALARM POINT	OIL	EMOTION
PERICARDIUM	Humility	Not Good Enough
PERIOSTEUM	Melrose	Injury
PERIOSTEUM	Present Time	Flustered
PERITONEUM	Onycha *or* Sandalwood	Terror
PEYER'S PATCHES	Ginger	Lack
PHYSICAL BODY	Valor	Losing a Battle
PINEAL	Sacred Mountain	Fear of the Unknown
PINEAL	Valor	Withdrawn
PITUITARY	Vetiver	Purpose *(Not fulfilling)*
PITUITARY	Ylang Ylang	Fear of Wisdom
PLEURA	Eucalyptus	Physical Stress
PLEURA	Lemon	Suffocated
PLEURA	Release	Dejection
PONS	Dorado Azuil *or* Forgiveness	Revenge
PONS	Jasmine	Feeling Unworthy
POSTERIOR FONTANEL	Marjoram	Unfulfilled
PSIS	Legacy *or* Myrrh	Difficulty
RAPHE NUCLEUS	Lavendar	Fear of Unfoldment
RAPHE NUCLEUS	Marjoram	Suspicious
RECTUM	Present Time	Resistance to Change
RETICULAR ACTIVATING SYSTEM	Oregano	Vunerable
RNA	Inner Child	Desertion
RNA	Live with Passion	Pushing
ROOF OF MOUTH	Brain Power *or* GeneYus	Brain Fog
SACRAL DOOR	Awaken	Connecting Interdimensionally
SALIVA GLANDS	Thieves	Uncertain
SEMINAL VESICLES/ FALLOPIAN TUBES	Harmony	Fear of Punishment *or* Beating Self Up
SENSORY PERCEPTION	Hope	Lack of Respect
SIGMOID COLON	Present Time	Repressed *or* Stuffed Emotions
SINUS	Lemon	Stuck

ALARM POINT	OIL	EMOTION
SKIN	Lavendar	Criticism
SKIN	Magnify Your Purpose	Humiliation
SMALL INTESTINE	Cinnamon Bark	Phony
SMALL INTESTINE	Lavender	Abandonment
SMALL INTESTINE	Transformation	Cynicism
SOLAR PLEXUS	Acceptance	Don't Belong
SOLAR PLEXUS	Exodus II	Doomed
SOLAR PLEXUS	Joy	Judgment
SOLAR PLEXUS – 3rd Chakra	Sacred Mountain	Being a part of Mass Consciousness
SOLAR PLEXUS	Transformation	Trapped (*Feeling*)
SOLAR PLEXUS	White Angelica	Sympathy
SOUL	Sacred Mountain	Compromising Self
SOUL (C2)	German Chamomile	Disassociation
SOUL INTEGRATION	Awaken	Expansion
SOURCE	Grounding	Lost
SPINAL CORD	Citronella	Wishy-Washy
SPINAL CORD	Copaiba	Lies
SPINAL CORD	Lemon	Fear of Detachment
SPLEEN	Believe	Dishonesty
SPLEEN	Clarity	Guilt
SPLEEN	Ledum	Ungrateful
STAPH	Purification	Being Alone
STOMACH	Chivalry *or* Harmony	Stubborn
STOMACH	Copaiba	Not Getting Enough
STOMACH	Peace & Calming	Losing Control
STOMACH	Valor	Defensiveness
STREP	Harmony	Being Ignored
3rd EYE	Elemi	Diabolical Disorientation
3rd EYE	Palo Santo	Limbo
3rd EYE	Sandalwood	Fear

ALARM POINT	OIL	EMOTION
TEMPORAL BONE/ MASTOID PORTION	Pepper, Black	Being in a Black Hole
TEMPORAL BONE/ MASTOID PORTION	Rosewood	Blindsided
TENDON	Lemongrass	Should
TESTES/OVARIES	Clarity	Fear of Repression
THALAMUS	Peppermint	Fear of Dependence
THALAMUS	Tea Tree	Stupid
THROAT	Sacred Mountain	Fear of Speaking Out
THROAT	Palo Santo	Obliteration
THYMUS	Peppermint	Failure
THYROID	Highest Potential	Get Even
THYROID	Peace & Calming	Argumentiveness
THYROID	Sacred Mountain	Injustice
TMJ	Present Time	Loss
TONGUE	Clove	Lashing Out
TONSIL	Lemon	Regret/Remorse *(Self-blame)*
TOXIC	Clary Sage	Intolerance *(General)*
TOXIC	JuvaFlex	Blame
TRACHEA	Release	Holding Back *(Universal flow)*
TRANSVERSE FIBERS	White Angelica	Resolution
UNCONSCIOUS	Aroma Siez	Fear of Inconsistency
UNCONSCIOUS	Lemon	Fear of Life Being Unreliable
UTERUS/PROSTATE	Forgiveness	Distrust
UTERUS/PROSTATE	Release	Loss of Identity
VEINS	Cypress	Disrespect
VERTEX – 8th Chakra	Idaho Balsam Fir	Separate
VERTEX – 7th Chakra	Release	Rebellion
VIBRATION	Longevity	Choked
VIRUS	Present Time	Illusion
VIRUS	Rose	Disintegrated

ALARM POINT	OIL	EMOTION
VIRUS	Transformation	Can't
VISION	EndoFlex	Denial
VISION	Envision	Attachment
VISION	Envision	Overwhelmed
VISION	Geranium	Self-Centered
VISION	Lime	Belittled
VOCAL CORDS	Tansy, Idaho	Misunderstood
WHITE BLOOD CELLS	Pine	Degraded
WHITE BLOOD CELLS	Valor	Inability to Cope
WILL @ C-5	Western or Canadian Red Cedar or Cedarwood	Incompletion
WILL @ C-5	Cassia	Dependent
YEAST/UMBILICUS	En-R-Gee	Connection
YEAST/UMBILICUS	Marjoram	Disconnected

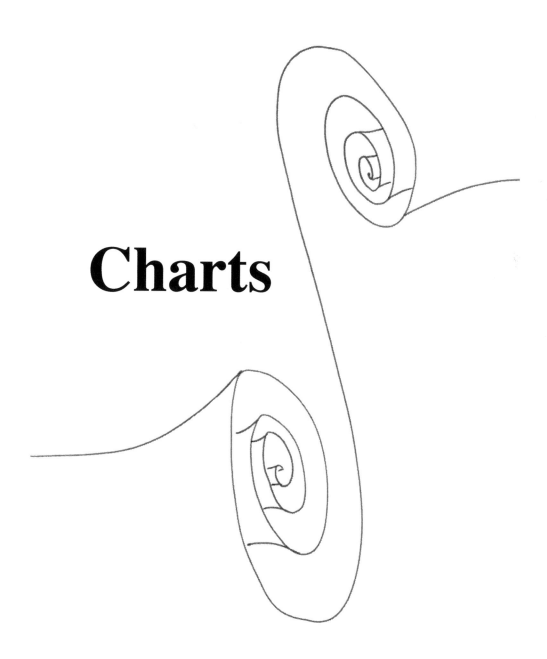

Charts

LOCATION OF BODY ALARM POINTS

All points are located and treated on both sides of the body unless found on the midline.

ALARM POINT	LOCATION	CHART
Accessory Spleen	1" anterior to Spleen	D
Adenoids	Simultaneous contact on nasal bone	A, B, D
Adrenal	2" superior & lateral to umbilicus @ 45 degrees	D, G, H
Adrenal Cortex	Midway between ribs & ASIS (top of hip bone—front of body)	D
Allergy	Right side, midway between nipple and xyphoid at 6th or 7th intercostal space	C
Amygdala	At hairline above middle of eye	A, C
Anterior Fontanel	Top of head @ midline behind frontal bone (GV-22)	B
Aorta	Episternal notch, CV-22 just above sternum on midline	A, C
Appendix	Right side, midway between ASIS & Umbilicus	D, H
Arteries	Middle of Sternocleidomastoidious (SCM, neck muscle)	B, D
Bacteria	1" above Umbilicus	D
Bladder	Midline, 3" above symphysis pubis (junction of pubis)	C, E, G, H
Blood	Lateral to breast in line with nipples	C
Blood Pressure	Middle of Biceps	E
Bone	Center of sacrum on midline	F
Bone Marrow	Junction of manibrum (upper 3 inches) & body of sternum	D
Bones of Ear	Behind ear cartilage in line with ear canal	B
Brain	Midline at hairline (GV-24)	A, B, E, G, H
Brain Integration	1" above center of top of ear	B, F
Breast	Upper medial quadrant @ 45 degree angle from nipple on breast tissue	D, E
Bronchial	2" above nipple, just lateral to sternum	C, G
C1	Lateral to atlas @ C1	B, F
Capillary	Level with bottom of ribs, 2" lateral to midline	D
Cellular Memory	1" above Bacteria	D, H

ALARM POINT	LOCATION	CHART
Cerebral Spinal Fluid	Head, on midline between Vertex and Posterior Fontanel (GV-19)	B, F
Cervix/Penis	1" above Symphysis Pubis	C
Chi	2" below Umbilicus midline (below Virus)	E
CNS/Lymph (Central Nerv. System)	Chin and neck junction on midline	A, B, C
Common Bile Duct	On side in line with Gallbladder and Pancreas	C, H
Connector	Behind the upper end of SCM (Sternocleidomastoid Muscle)	B
Courage	3" superior & 1" lateral to Umbilicus	E
Creativity	1" medial & 1" superior to medial spine of scapula	F
CX @ CV-5 Circulation/Sex	1" above Bladder alarm (CX @ CV-5)	C, E
Depression	1" above mastoid portion of temporal bone	B
Diaphragm	3" bilaterally along Cartilage of ribs, starting at sternum	C, G
Disc	Immediately inferior to lateral clavicle above Lung alarm	D
DNA	Ear lobe	B
Duodenum	Lower border of 11th rib 2" lateral to nipple	E
Ear, Bones of	Behind ear cartilage in line with ear canal	B
Ear, External	Over cartilage of ear	B
Ear, Inner	Over ear canal	B, H
Ear, Middle	Immediately above the Tragus	B
Ego	1" below xyphoid (bottom of sternum)	E
Emotional Integration	Between supraorbital notch & Thalamus	A, B, E
Emotional Point	Frontal eminence	A
Energy Channel	2" medial to ASIS	C
Epiglottis	Bilateral 1" lateral & 1" inferior to Laryngeal Prominence	A, B, D
Esophagus	1" below nipple near sternum	E, G
Eustachian	Tube Front of ear immediately below tragus	B, G
External Ear	Over Cartilage of ear	B
Eye	Center of eye lid, apply oil on hand or feet eye points only	G, H

ALARM POINT	LOCATION	CHART
Eye/Brain On Occiput	2" behind back center of ear	B, F
Eye Lymph	Lateral & inferior to lateral corner of eye on bone	A
Eye on Parietal	1" lateral to Anterior Fontanel	B
Eye, 3rd	Midline just above eyebrows between Hypothalamus & Sinus	A, E
Fascia	Greater trocanter of femur (top of leg)	E, H
Fallopian Tubes/ Seminal Vesicles	1" lateral & superior to lateral border of pubis	C
Filter	1" lateral to Spinal Cord & 1" above on occiput	B, F
First Rib	Neck & shoulder junction on side of body	C, F
Fontanel, Anterior	Top of head @ midline behind frontal bone	B
Fontanel, Posterior	Midline back of head above occipital bone	B
Fungus	Center of lower medial quadrant of breast (1" below & 1" lateral to Stomach alarm)	E
Gallbladder	Inferior to nipple under breast on right side	C, G, H
Gums/Teeth	Center of maxillary, under cheek bone	B, E
GV-20	Top of head, midline above ear	B, F
Hara	2" below Xyphoid (bottom of Sternum)	D
Harmony	1" superior to medial spine of scapula (WBC)	F
Head of Pancreas	Left side 1/2" lateral & 2" inferior to Stomach	C, E
Heart	Mandible, midway between angle of jaw and chin	B, G, H
Heart Center	3" superior & 2" lateral to Stomach alarm	E
Heart Constrictor	Middle of body of sternum	C
Heart Protector	2" inferior to middle of Clavicle	D
Heart Strings	2" above Nipple of Breast	D
Heavy Metals	Anterior Superior Iliac Spine	E
Hepatic Duct	Right side, between 7th & 8th Ribs	E
Higher Will	Behind SCM Lateral to C3	B, F
Hippocampus	Supraorbital Notch (Upper Medial Eye)	A, C

ALARM POINT	LOCATION	CHART
Hormone	Midline, center of nose, junction of nasal bone & cartilage	A, E
Hypothalamus	Between eyebrows, above nose, below 3rd Eye	A, E
ICV - Ileocecal Valve	Phylum on midline between nose and upper lip	A, E, G
Ileum	10th rib on side	E
Immune	1" lateral to Lymph on lateral upper chest	C
Infection	1/2" lateral to Vertex	B, F
Injury	Space just medial to junction of lateral Clavicle and Scapula on top of shoulder.	E, F
Innocence	Center of Eye between Eye and Supraorbital bone	A. B
Integration @ L3	2" lateral to L3	F
Inner Ear	Over ear canal	B, H
Intuitive	2" below & 2" lateral to Medial Clavicular Head	E
Joints/Cartilage	2nd intercostal space next to sternum	E
Kidney	1" superior & lateral to Umbilicus @ 45 degree angle	D, G, H
Large Intestine	1" inferior & lateral to Umbilicus @ 45 degree angle	D, G, H
Laryngeal Prominence	Adam's apple	A, C
Larynx	1" below Chin/neck Junction on Midline	A, C
Life Force	Spinous Process of L3	F
Ligament	Sacroiliac Ligament @ upper junction of hip & sacrum	F, H
Liver	Nipple of breast	C, D, G, H
Locus Ceruleus (Brain Immune System)	1/2" lateral & inferior to occipital protuberance	B, F
Lung	1" inferior to lateral clavicle & 1" medial to humerous @ LU-1	C, G, H
Lymph	Midway between Lung & Liver (Lateral Chest) (nipple)	C
Lymphatic Congestion	Lower lateral corner of breast	C
Lymph Valves	Angle of lower ribs on inferior border 1" medial to nipple line	C
Magic	1" lateral to Umbilicus	C

ALARM POINT	LOCATION	CHART
Mastoid Portion of Temporal Bone	Behind jaw below the ear	B
Medulla	2" lateral to midline between Pineal & Spinal Cord	B, F
Meninges	Parietal Eminence 2" superior and 3" lateral to Posterior Fontanel	B, F
Middle Ear	Immediately above the Tragus	B
Mold	Center of lower lateral Quadrant of breast (45° from nipple)	D
Mucous Membranes	End of nose	A, C
Muscle	L5 & S1 junction	F
Nerve	3" superior to medial end of spine of scapula on top of shoulder (Top of shoulders between neck and shoulder)	C, D, F
Nerve Root	2" below and 1" lateral to medial clavicular head	E
Ovaries	1" medial to ASIS	C
Pancreas	Left side below breast in line with nipple	C, G, H
Pancreas, Head of	Left side 1/2" lateral & 2" inferior to Stomach	C, E
Pancreatic Duct	Left side 3" inferior & 2" medial to nipple	E
Parasites	Middle of right Groin on Inguinal ligament	D
Parathyroid	1" lateral to Laryngeal Prominence or Adam's apple	A, B, D, G, H
Parotid	Below angle of jaw under mandible	B
Pericardium	1" superior to nipple lateral to sternum	E
Periosteum	Middle of dorsal surface back of Hand	H
Peritoneum	2" above symphysis pubis (junction of pubis) on midline	C
Peyer's Patches	1" lateral & superior to Lymph valves on lower rib	D
Physical Body	Midline below lower lip	A
Pineal	Occipital protuberance (GV-16)	B, F, H
Pituitary	Above eyebrows, anterior on right, posterior on left	A, E, G, H
Pleura	Anterior axilla under pectoral muscle	C
Pons	Midway between Anterior Fontanel & hairline on midline (GV-23)	A, B, D
Posterior Fontanel	Midline back of head above occipital bone (GV-17)	B, F
PSIS	Posterior Superior Iliac Spine	F

ALARM POINT	LOCATION	CHART
Raphe Nucleus	Above Posterior Fontanel on midline (GV-18)	B, F
Rectum	Left side, midway betweeen ASIS & pubis	E, G
Reticular Activating System	1" lateral & 1" superior to Posterior Fontanel	B, F
RNA	1" lateral between Posterior Fontanel and Pineal	B, F
Roof of Mouth	Place tip of tongue or thumb on center of Roof of Mouth or suck thumb for Brain alignment	Not on chart
Sacral Door	Double contact, 1" inferior & 1" lateral to top of sacrum	F
Saliva Glands	Behind the jaw on neck below ear behind ear lobe	B
Seminal Vesicles/ Fallopian Tubes	Fallopian Tubes 1" lateral & superior to lateral border of pubis	C
Sensory Perception	Upper outer corner above eye, below eyebrow	A
Sigmoid Colon	Midway between ASIS & Umbilicus on left side	E, G
Sinus	Midline @ center of forehead 1" above 3rd Eye	A, E, G, H
Skin	End of 12th rib	F
Small Intestine	Midway between last rib & ASIS @ waist	E, F, G, H
Solar Plexus	3" below xyphoid or midline	D, G
Soul	Lateral to & between C2 & C3	B, F
Soul Integration	1" anterior & 1" above center of top of ear	B
Source	Between muscle & bone on sacrum space between S1 & S2 on midline	F
Spinal Cord	Base of occiput at neck & head junction (GV-15)	B, F, H
Spleen, Accessory	1" anterior to Spleen	D
Spleen	2" above lower edge of ribs on side	D, G, H
Staph	Top of SCM muscle, 1" below ear on neck	B
Stomach	Near sternum medial to nipple	C, E, G, H
Strep	Above middle of clavicle (on collar bone)	A, C
3rd Eye	Midline just above eyebrows between Hypothalamus & Sinus	A, E
Temporal Bone, Mastoid Portion	Behind jaw below the ear	B

ALARM POINT	LOCATION	CHART
Tendon	Lateral to Spinal Cord along base of occiput	B, F
Testes	Upper, inner thigh	C
Thalamus	Lacrimal bone @ sides of nasal bone	A, B, E
Throat	Laryngeal Prominence (Adam's apple)	A
Thymus	Inferior to clavicle, lateral to manibrum @ K-27	A, C
Thyroid	Just above medial head of clavicle	A, C, G, H
TMJ	Anterior mandible under maxilla 1" lateral & inferior to cheek bone on maxilla	B
Tongue	Upper 1/3 of SCM – Anterior Border	B
Tonsil	Under chin midway between center and angle of jaw	B, D, H
Toxic	2" below nipple near sternum	E
Trachea	Midline below at bottom of Larynx 1" below Laryngeal Prominence (Adam's Apple)	A, B, C
Transverse Fibers	Top of cartilage of ear	B, F
Unconscious	Temple at sphenoid	B, D
Uterus/Prostate	Midline on symphysis pubis (Pubic Bone)	C
Veins	1" above xyphoid on midline of sternum	D
Vertex	Midline @ top of skull between fontanels (GV-21)	B, C, F
Vibration	End of Xyphoid	D
Virus	1" below Umbilicus	D, E, H
Vision	Center of temple 1" above zygomatic arch	B
Vocal Cords	Bilateral 1" above Parathyroid lateral to Laryngeal Prominence	A, B, C
White Blood Cells	Medial end of spine of scapula	F
Will @ C-5	Lateral to C-5	B, F
Yeast/Umbilicus	Navel	C, D

NOTE: 1" refers to the human inch which is the distance
between the first and second joint of the index finger.
Most points are approximately the size of a quarter.
While you want to be as precise as possible, you
do have some leeway.

CHART A

FACE - Front

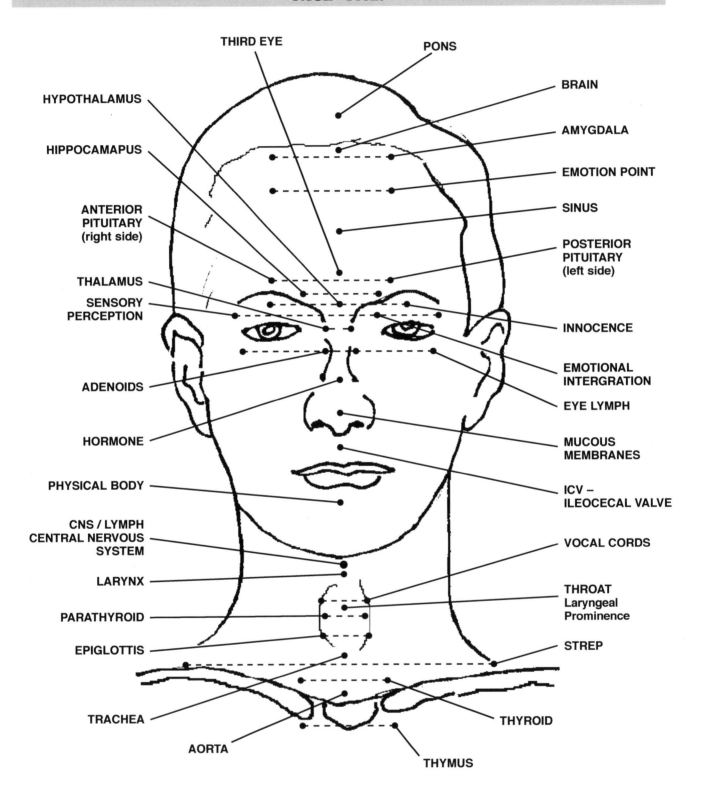

THIRD EYE

PONS

BRAIN

HYPOTHALAMUS

AMYGDALA

HIPPOCAMAPUS

EMOTION POINT

ANTERIOR
PITUITARY
(right side)

SINUS

POSTERIOR
PITUITARY
(left side)

THALAMUS

SENSORY
PERCEPTION

INNOCENCE

EMOTIONAL
INTERGRATION

ADENOIDS

EYE LYMPH

HORMONE

MUCOUS
MEMBRANES

PHYSICAL BODY

ICV –
ILEOCECAL VALVE

CNS / LYMPH
CENTRAL NERVOUS
SYSTEM

VOCAL CORDS

LARYNX

THROAT
Laryngeal
Prominence

PARATHYROID

EPIGLOTTIS

STREP

TRACHEA

THYROID

AORTA

THYMUS

CHART B

FACE - Side

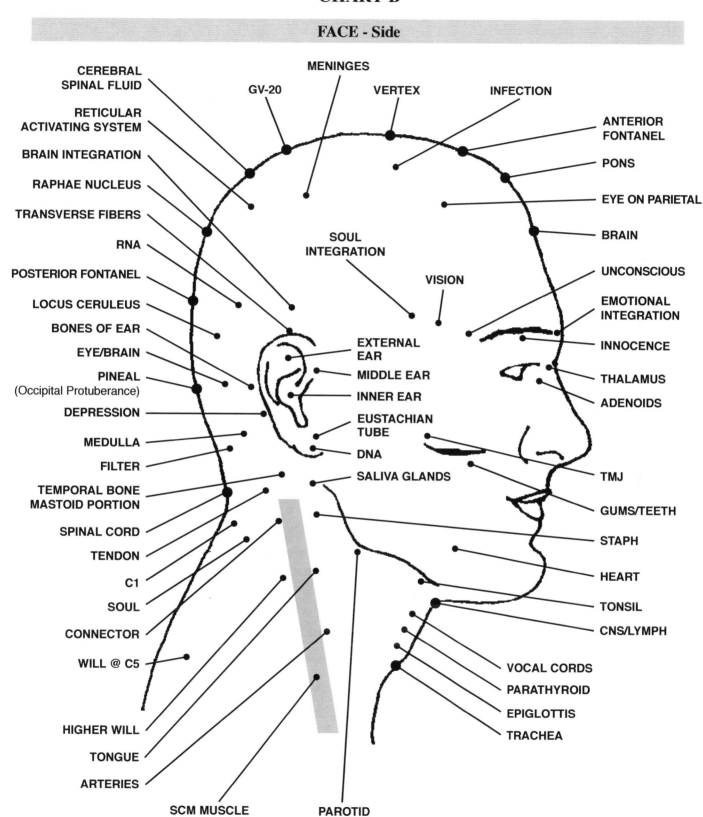

CEREBRAL SPINAL FLUID

RETICULAR ACTIVATING SYSTEM

BRAIN INTEGRATION

RAPHAE NUCLEUS

TRANSVERSE FIBERS

RNA

POSTERIOR FONTANEL

LOCUS CERULEUS

BONES OF EAR

EYE/BRAIN

PINEAL
(Occipital Protuberance)

DEPRESSION

MEDULLA

FILTER

TEMPORAL BONE MASTOID PORTION

SPINAL CORD

TENDON

C1

SOUL

CONNECTOR

WILL @ C5

HIGHER WILL

TONGUE

ARTERIES

MENINGES

GV-20

VERTEX

INFECTION

SOUL INTEGRATION

VISION

EXTERNAL EAR

MIDDLE EAR

INNER EAR

EUSTACHIAN TUBE

DNA

SALIVA GLANDS

ANTERIOR FONTANEL

PONS

EYE ON PARIETAL

BRAIN

UNCONSCIOUS

EMOTIONAL INTEGRATION

INNOCENCE

THALAMUS

ADENOIDS

TMJ

GUMS/TEETH

STAPH

HEART

TONSIL

CNS/LYMPH

VOCAL CORDS

PARATHYROID

EPIGLOTTIS

TRACHEA

SCM MUSCLE

PAROTID

CHART C

Front Torso 1

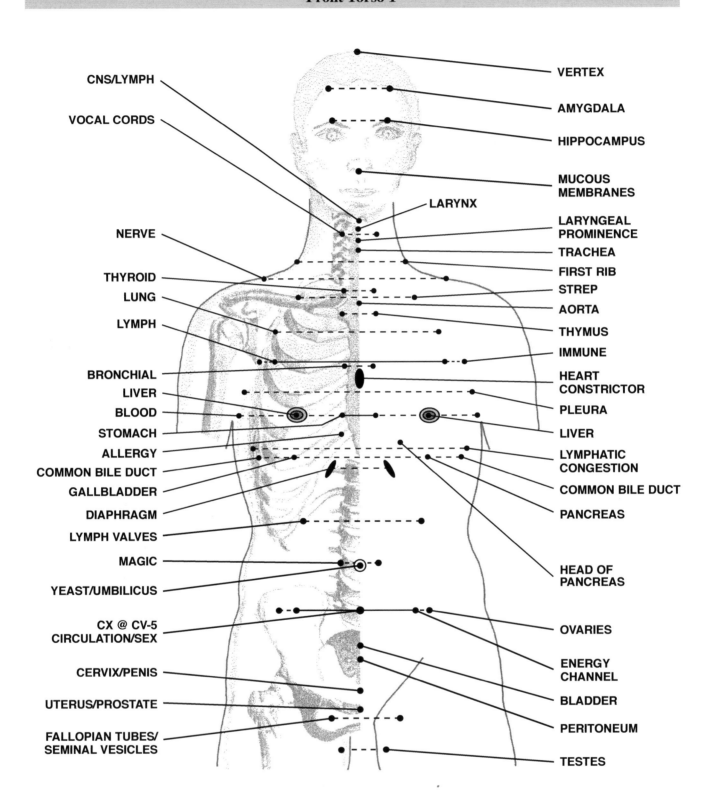

CNS/LYMPH

VOCAL CORDS

NERVE

THYROID

LUNG

LYMPH

BRONCHIAL

LIVER

BLOOD

STOMACH

ALLERGY

COMMON BILE DUCT

GALLBLADDER

DIAPHRAGM

LYMPH VALVES

MAGIC

YEAST/UMBILICUS

CX @ CV-5
CIRCULATION/SEX

CERVIX/PENIS

UTERUS/PROSTATE

FALLOPIAN TUBES/
SEMINAL VESICLES

VERTEX

AMYGDALA

HIPPOCAMPUS

MUCOUS
MEMBRANES

LARYNX

LARYNGEAL
PROMINENCE

TRACHEA

FIRST RIB

STREP

AORTA

THYMUS

IMMUNE

HEART
CONSTRICTOR

PLEURA

LIVER

LYMPHATIC
CONGESTION

COMMON BILE DUCT

PANCREAS

HEAD OF
PANCREAS

OVARIES

ENERGY
CHANNEL

BLADDER

PERITONEUM

TESTES

CHART D

Front Torso 2

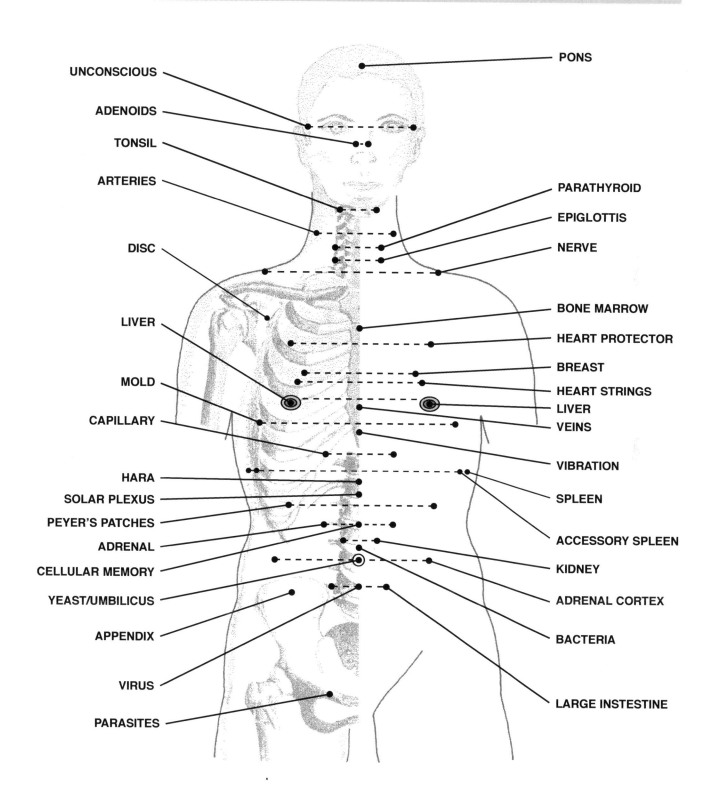

PONS
UNCONSCIOUS
ADENOIDS
TONSIL
ARTERIES
PARATHYROID
EPIGLOTTIS
NERVE
DISC
BONE MARROW
LIVER
HEART PROTECTOR
BREAST
MOLD
HEART STRINGS
LIVER
CAPILLARY
VEINS
VIBRATION
HARA
SOLAR PLEXUS
SPLEEN
PEYER'S PATCHES
ADRENAL
ACCESSORY SPLEEN
CELLULAR MEMORY
KIDNEY
YEAST/UMBILICUS
ADRENAL CORTEX
APPENDIX
BACTERIA
VIRUS
LARGE INSTESTINE
PARASITES

CHART E

Front Torso 3

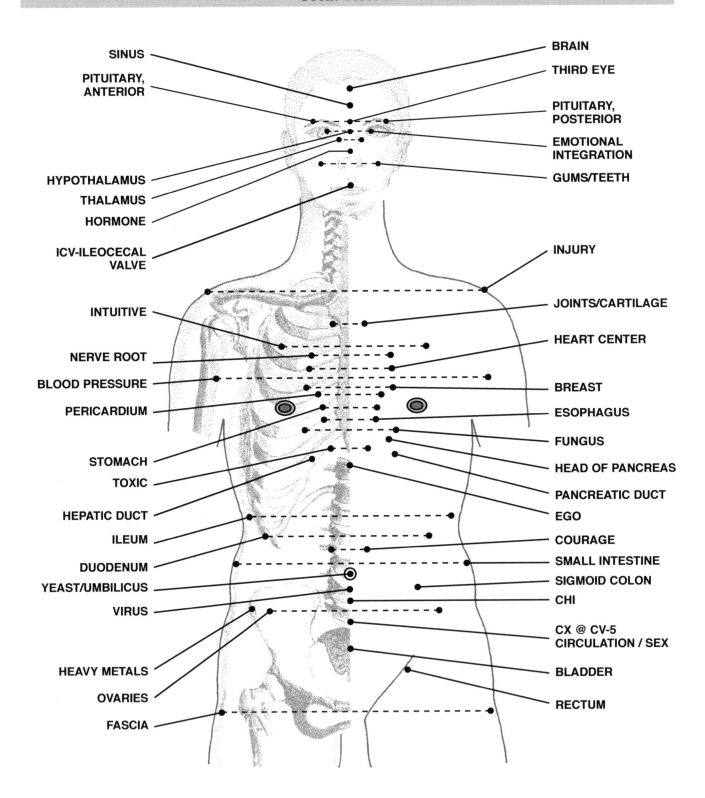

SINUS

PITUITARY,
ANTERIOR

HYPOTHALAMUS

THALAMUS

HORMONE

ICV-ILEOCECAL
VALVE

INTUITIVE

NERVE ROOT

BLOOD PRESSURE

PERICARDIUM

STOMACH

TOXIC

HEPATIC DUCT

ILEUM

DUODENUM

YEAST/UMBILICUS

VIRUS

HEAVY METALS

OVARIES

FASCIA

BRAIN

THIRD EYE

PITUITARY,
POSTERIOR

EMOTIONAL
INTEGRATION

GUMS/TEETH

INJURY

JOINTS/CARTILAGE

HEART CENTER

BREAST

ESOPHAGUS

FUNGUS

HEAD OF PANCREAS

PANCREATIC DUCT

EGO

COURAGE

SMALL INTESTINE

SIGMOID COLON

CHI

CX @ CV-5
CIRCULATION / SEX

BLADDER

RECTUM

CHART F

Back Torso

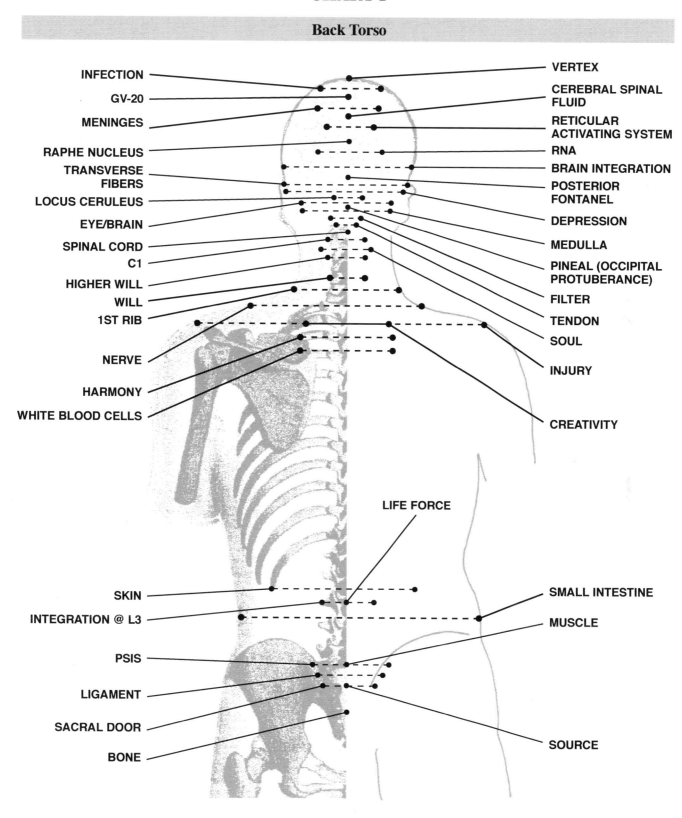

INFECTION

GV-20

MENINGES

RAPHE NUCLEUS

TRANSVERSE FIBERS

LOCUS CERULEUS

EYE/BRAIN

SPINAL CORD

C1

HIGHER WILL

WILL

1ST RIB

NERVE

HARMONY

WHITE BLOOD CELLS

VERTEX

CEREBRAL SPINAL FLUID

RETICULAR ACTIVATING SYSTEM

RNA

BRAIN INTEGRATION

POSTERIOR FONTANEL

DEPRESSION

MEDULLA

PINEAL (OCCIPITAL PROTUBERANCE)

FILTER

TENDON

SOUL

INJURY

CREATIVITY

LIFE FORCE

SKIN

INTEGRATION @ L3

PSIS

LIGAMENT

SACRAL DOOR

BONE

SMALL INTESTINE

MUSCLE

SOURCE

CHART G

Foot Reflex Points

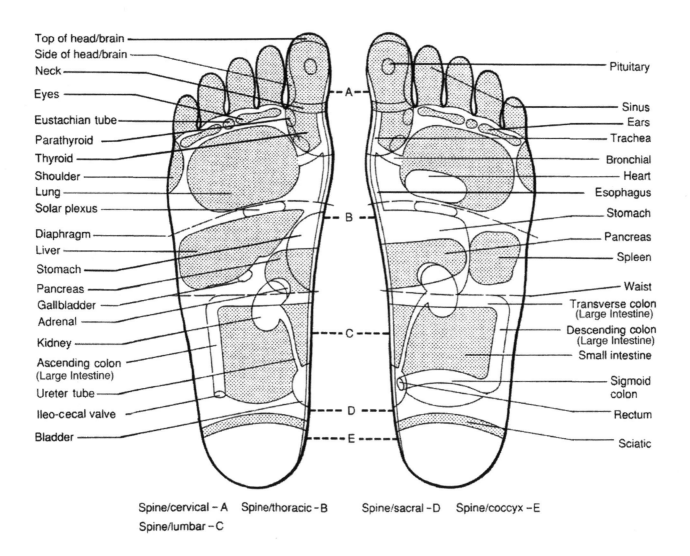

Top of head/brain
Side of head/brain
Neck
Eyes
Eustachian tube
Parathyroid
Thyroid
Shoulder
Lung
Solar plexus
Diaphragm
Liver
Stomach
Pancreas
Gallbladder
Adrenal
Kidney
Ascending colon (Large Intestine)
Ureter tube
Ileo-cecal valve
Bladder

Pituitary
Sinus
Ears
Trachea
Bronchial
Heart
Esophagus
Stomach
Pancreas
Spleen
Waist
Transverse colon (Large Intestine)
Descending colon (Large Intestine)
Small intestine
Sigmoid colon
Rectum
Sciatic

Spine/cervical – A   Spine/thoracic – B   Spine/sacral – D   Spine/coccyx – E
Spine/lumbar – C

Oils may be applied only to the feet, used on the Body Alarm Points, or on both areas to treat a specific organ or area.

CHART H

ALTERNATIVES FOR HARD TO ACCESS POINTS

Since some of the body alarm points are hard to access in public, like the liver point, you may wish to use the hand points when you are working on clearing deep-seated patterns that you want to treat frequently. Occasionally there may be times when a point on the body or feet is extremely sensitive, treating it on the hands is equally effective. Reflex points on the hands and feet may be used in addition to, or instead of those on the body. Treat the points on both hands even though they may only be shown on one hand.

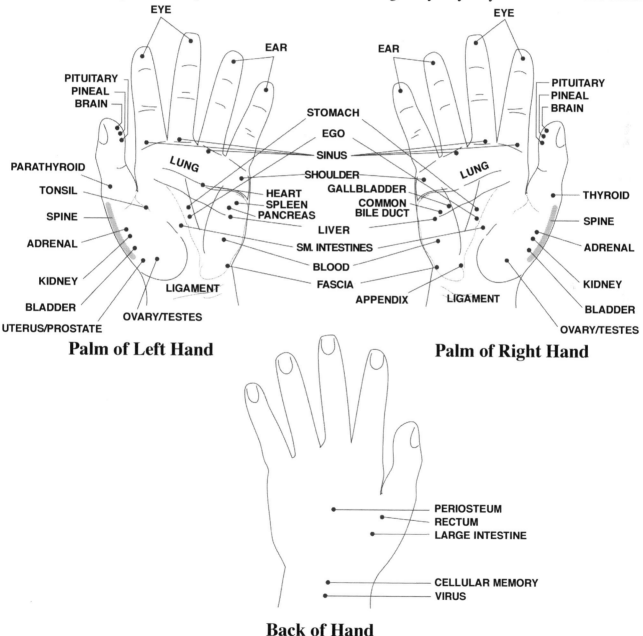

Palm of Left Hand   **Palm of Right Hand**

Back of Hand

Clearing
Enhancements

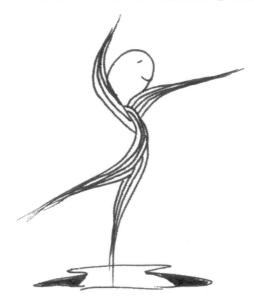

DISCOVERING ADDITIONAL EMOTIONAL PATTERNS

Now that you know how to clear obvious emotions that surface, you can begin to look at some of the emotions that surround a major or core issue. A core issue is an issue that carries significant disruptive energy. It has usually been in operation a long time and is easy to recognize. Examples of core issues are rejection, abandonment, anger, and control.

Working With Core Issues & Their Tentacles

The easiest way to find and distinguish core issues and their related tentacles is to observe your pattern of reaction. When you find yourself upset at someone or some situation, you are probably reacting to the person or situation with a conditioned response. A conditioned response could look something like yelling, storming out of the room, simply closing down to the person, or leaving the situation.

The way to identify your emotions and issues is to observe your conditioned response. Whenever you find yourself reacting, look to see what you are feeling.

You have probably noticed that when certain situations come up, like someone having an opinion that is different from yours, you feel bad. When you are able to go within yourself and check it out, by being aware of where the feeling is located in your body or what thoughts arise when you ask yourself what is going on, rejection comes up. You have just identified your core emotional pattern.

Let's say you have been working on releasing rejection for a few days and you encounter a similar situation of someone else with a different opinion than yours. Perhaps this time it was a more forceful energy and subconsciously you felt threatened. Your immediate response would be to react, which relates to the emotion of conflict. Along with conflict is the need to control in order to protect and feel safe. Once out of the immediate perceived danger, the feeling of betrayal surfaces, then disrespect or blame. Once the hurt subsides, up comes rejection again, then victim. Knowing you can't function in the world in this weakened, vulnerable state, up comes F—You. When nothing seems to work, you are left with the feeling of failure.

Rejection

(core issue/emotion)

Threatened   Conflict   Control

Betrayal

Disrespect/Blame

Hurt — Rejection

Victim

F–You

Failure

These are some of the most common related emotions, Check to see which one(s) are present for you. Working on several emotions simultaneously reduces the emotional charge much faster than just working on the core issue.

The Tentacles of Control

The purpose of the ego is to keep us safe, and one of its main defenses is control. All control is based on fear. Therefore, we all have control issues to some degree. We control by controlling ourselves, others, and/or our environment. To determine whether control is an emotion you currently need to address, ask yourself, "Do you have a fear of being controlled? Or do you have a need to be in control? Or both?" Most people experience both the need to control and the fear of being controlled. However, one is normally more dominant than the other.

Fear of being Controlled

Fear of being controlled can appear as a need to work alone, be your own boss, or having difficulty playing on a team. Even following a schedule, especially someone else's, can bring up fear of being controlled.

Anyone who has been hurt in a controlled environment, as a child or adult, could develop the "fear of being controlled" as a core issue.

Emotions that are connected to fear of being controlled are fear of authority, confined, dependence, disrespect, domineering, restriction, and suppression.

If you have the core issue "fear of being controlled" you would be triggered by any situation remotely similar to the time you were hurt. Your "reaction" to authority may be out of proportion to the current reality and you may see someone as domineering when they are simply being strong. This "triggered" response applies to any and all of the emotions connected to control.

Avoiding structure at home or work could be indicative of "fear of being controlled." Can you view structure as a supportive tool that enables you to achieve balance in your life? If you have very little structure in your life, you may wish to check in and see if "fear of control" is in operation.

Even setting your own structure can trigger "fear of being controlled". Any structure, even your own, can trigger feeling confined, dominated, restricted or suppressed.

Needing to be in Control

The need to be in control can stem from "fear of being controlled". One way to avoid being controlled is to be in control at all times. If this applies to you, refer to "fear of being controlled" above.

The "need to be in control" usually appears as the need to have things done a certain way, your way. It is more to control the outcome, get things done right, on time, and successfully.

Children whose needs were not met due to incompetence by adults may develop "need to be in control" as a core issue. There may be an underlying belief that "the only way to get my needs met is to do it myself".

Emotions that are connected to "need to be in control" are distrust of authority, dependence, ignored, sabotage and unsupported.

If you have the core issue "need to be in control" you probably have become adept at doing everything you perceive you need in order to survive. You will most likely view other people, in general, as incompetent. By releasing the pattern "need to be in control" you will be able to relate to people according to who they are as a whole instead of whether or not they are competent in a specific area.

Control issues, both needing to be in control or fear of being controlled, can hinder or destroy marriages, friendships, business relationships or partnerships of any nature. Imagine trying to live or work together if one person has "fear of being controlled" and the other has "need to control." Everything they would do or say would "trigger" the other. Now imagine both people releasing their patterns. The love and/or respect they have for each other would be free to be expressed and the relationship would be able to develop into something dynamic that would have been impossible with both people operating in the "control" issues.

Survival Issues

Basic survival issues include the "fear of losing," which triggers memories stored in the cellular memory of losing one's life whenever a battle was lost. The fear of losing is triggered anytime you find yourself in a conflict or disagreement with someone else. Past experience usually relates to losing something, like a business or a friendship, whenever there is conflict. The solution is to change the rules of the game from a "win/lose" to one of mutual growth. This means both parties can win.

The fear of being wrong relates to losing face, to not being good enough, to losing, and failure. All of these are really opportunities for growth and coming from your place of knowingness. It's our challenges that show us our weak areas and point us in the direction we need to go.

Some emotions, like betrayal, bring denied thoughts and feelings into conscious awareness. The other side of betrayal is faithfulness, which ultimately means being faithful to ourselves. Since our outer world reflects what is going on inside of us, being betrayed by someone else occurs after we have betrayed a part of ourselves. "I have the courage to accept the truth" commands the truth to reveal itself. This allows the underlying fears, like fear of failure or conflict, to surface. As soon as these emotions are recognized, they can be cleared. As a result, you can add more oils, meaning you will be working with a number of emotional patterns simultaneously.

When you face powerful issues like betrayal, your life can change because the parts of you that have been denied will surface. These are the parts you can no longer ignore. Be aware that they would not present themselves until you have the tools to be able to handle them. So even though the clearing process can be challenging, the outcome or reward is positive, often better than you could have imagined.

General Clearing

We live in a toxic environment. Our air and water are polluted. Between our computers and cell phones we are constantly bombarded with electromagnetic stress. Our foods are full of chemicals and preservatives. We are exposed to chemicals on a daily basis. Since we live in a world of duality, I knew there had to be a positive side to toxicity. Why else would it be on the increase? In addition to the toxins in our environment, we create our own stress every time we allow ourselves to get into a negative emotional state.

When we experience negative emotions, it reinforces or creates an emotional pattern. We feel the energy first in the center of our body in our abdomen or chest region. The feeling then goes to the head affecting the hormonal system.

Then the digestive system shuts down, which in turn causes all the food in the intestines to putrefy, resulting in a toxic bowel. The oil *Legacy* affects the lower body including the elimination system.

The other side of toxicity is transformation. Transformation relates to moving forward into a higher state of consciousness. The way out is by going "into the void" which corresponds to going into the eye of the hurricane, or passing through the eye of the needle. It's going into the still small place within, slipping through the crack, the point where the infinity sign crosses. The oil is *Legacy* and the alarm point is the Connector located on the back side of the upper 1/3rd of the sternocleidomastoid muscle, which is between the ear and the spinal cord on the neck at the base of the skull.

As with all the clearing, you may wish to include the Release point at the top of the spine, and the Filter points on the back of the head.

The clearing effect is amazing. There is usually a release of blocked energy and clarity that appears in the eyes. The eyes are incredible; the life returns and they sparkle. The brain fog lifts; the life force floods through the body and there is a feeling of having energy. Clearing the toxicity often provides a sense of being grounded or solidly connected with the earth. A related emotion is difficulty. Difficulty relates to life's challenges with the "other side" coming from a place of knowing.

**Recap for oil Legacy*:*
Feeling: Toxicity—environmental from food, air and water, electromagnetic, chemical, and emotional.
Other side: Transformation
Alarm point: Connector
Way out: "Into the void."

Emotion: Difficulty
Other Side: Knowing
Alarm Point: PSIS
Way Out: "I move with life."

The next oil is *Release* which affects the center of the body. Two of the most common negative emotions are fear of being wrong and fear of success. Fear of being wrong is located in the accessory spleen which lies in front of the spleen. The spleen is the major organ associated with the immune system. Chronic negative emotions will depress immune function. The emotion stored in the spleen is guilt. We feel guilty because we feel we have done something wrong.

Another common emotion you may wish to include is fear of success. The other side is rejection. If you are afraid of success, what do you get? Rejection. You feel more comfortable with rejection since this is what you know rather than with the unknown success. This leads to sabotage as a means of protection. If you refuse to accept success because you feel you don't deserve it or can't handle it, you are rejecting success. The way out is "I accept awareness."

Recap for oil Release

Emotion: Wrong (fear of being)

Emotion: Success (fear of)

Other Side: Knowingness

Other Side: Rejection

Alarm Point: Accessory Spleen

Alarm Point: Large Intestine

Way Out: "I am true to my Source."

Way Out: "I accept awareness."

Peppermint oil affects the head and throat. *Peppermint* is antibacterial, antifungal and antiviral as well as a good digestive aid. Associated emotions are restriction and failure. Restriction is stored in the medulla which is the area of the brain that controls both voluntary and involuntary muscles. Involuntary muscles control our heart beat, respiration and digestion. A related emotion is fear of failure. Failure is stored in the thymus which is part of the immune system. Adding *Peppermint* to your drinking water is very soothing to a sore throat. It will also improve the quality of the water. When adding *Peppermint* to your drinking water, start with one drop and increase according to desire. Get a large glass, fill it half full with water, add one drop *Peppermint* oil, fill the glass with water and drink throughout the day. As your glass gets empty, add more water. Some of the *Peppermint* oil will remain in the glass making adding more *Peppermint* an option.

Recap for oil Peppermint

Emotion: Restriction

Emotion: Failure

Other Side: Mobility

Other Side: Unfoldment

Alarm Point: Medulla

Alarm Point: Thymus

Way Out: "I am open to new experiences."

Way Out: "I accept growth."

PEACEFUL WARRIOR

We have been told that we are all connected, that we are all one. Yet, if this is true, why is there so much disharmony and misunderstanding? Wouldn't life be much simpler if everyone thought like we think? Practically speaking, not even families, partners, and loved ones live in perfect harmony. If we can't get along with people we deeply love, how can we be expected to live in harmony with people we don't even like? Yet every religion and spiritual teaching preaches love as the ultimate goal and the answer to all our problems. I found this to be an idealistic approach and very difficult to apply, especially when I found myself under attack. It was because of this dilemma that I wrote *Releasing Emotional Patterns with Essential Oils*. I felt we needed a bridge, a practical guide, to shift a negative feeling or experience into one that was love rather than fear-based.

Being a Thyroid body type, my strengths are Mental/Spiritual, so my way of dealing with emotions and uncomfortable situations is to first understand the situation (Mental) and then discover what I need to learn from it (Spiritual). I soon discovered that this was not enough. Since this is a planet of duality as illustrated by Einstein's theory of relativity, it stands to reason that emotions have both a negative (fear) and positive (love) expression. Consequently, when I experience someone being aggressive towards me, I have to look within to see what I have been doing or thinking that initiated my need to have this experience (taking personal responsibility, Spiritual). My next step is to access the higher octave or other side of the emotion (Mental), which, in this example of aggression, is respect. Then I feel (Emotional) both sides of the feelings in depth -- 3all the way to the core, allowing the feelings to express, even to the point of tears.

Now it is time to access the physical body. Emotions are stored in the cellular memory and reside in the organs or regions of the body that have a corresponding vibrational frequency, as well as in the limbic system of the brain. Contacting the emotional points on the forehead accesses the emotional pathway, smelling the appropriate oil, in this case *Valor,* and saying the affirmation or statement "I love", establishes a new pathway or bridge from aggression to respect. Applying the essential oil *Valor t*o the associated body alarm point, in this example adrenal cortex, releases cellular memory and allows me to choose a new way of being. It establishes a new pattern, so instead of reacting to the aggressive remark with aggression, I can respond from love and allow the other person to have their opinion, thus shifting or transmitting conflict into peace.

Astrologically, the planet Mars came closest to the earth on August 27, 2003, causing the qualities attributed to it to surface and become a focal point for humanity. Since the effect of Mars will be felt for the next 20 years, dealing with Mars energy is imperative. The attributes of Mars are: energy, movement, setting and meeting goals, getting things done quickly, impatience, war, and the need to communicate. Communication is the first step in conflict resolution and is essential in building a peaceful world.

Conflict resolution consists of four steps. The first is dialogue, which may be explosive and irrational nature. Often emotional, the words do not necessarily reflect the current triggering situation and carry with them a lot of past emotional baggage (karma). Once the situation or energy is on the table, it is time to look at the facts. This is an opportunity to determine what is real and what is illusion. The third step is questioning which requires taking an interest in the other person, walking in their shoes, seeing things from their perspective. The last step is debate; looking at both sides, examining the pros and cons of each to come up with a viable solution that meets the needs of both parties in a win win, not only for the present but the future as well. This solution is the spiritual aspect which corresponds to the lesson and is expressed in the statement under "Way Out" in the Emotional Reference section of this book.

Past cultures relied on priests, kings or judges to resolve conflict. We are now entering a time wherein everyone is required to master the art of resolution. In the 9th century, King Arthur's vision when he established the knights of the round table was to develop a new way of resolving conflict. The code of honor of a knight of the round table was to live at one's highest potential, transmuting the desire to get even into personal accomplishment and replacing annoyance with happiness. Doing chivalrous deeds was about intervening and ultimately empowering the powerless. Percival represents self-purification in the questioning process of asking the right question at the right time. The search for the Holy Grail is the process of becoming a free human being. Becoming a free human being requires releasing the old patterns that keep us locked in a negative behavior.

One of the best ways to identify negative patterns is to see what we are attracting in our relationships. Negative emotions are the most familiar and easiest to spot, providing an excellent entry point. Stress is the most common complaint and conflict is the number one cause. Conflict is held in the adrenal cortex and fear of facing the world in the adrenal glands. Becoming a peaceful warrior or knight of the round table where everyone is equally respected requires meeting conflict not with more conflict (war), but with peace. Peace requires meeting a negative response pattern with a higher frequency and operating from an internal place of peace.

I selected 12 essentials oils to be used along with the Chakra Harmony oils. The two Chakra Harmony oils I particularly like to include are Sacred Mountain and Idaho Balsam Fir. Sacred Mountain relates to the third Chakra at the solar plexus which is connected with being a part of mass consciousness. Idaho Balsam Fir is for the eighth Chakra which brings all the Chakras into balance and solidifies the intention to return body, mind and spirit to the point of perfection.

The Peaceful Warrior Travel Kit consists of 12 essential oils: Peace & Calming, Purification, Peppermint, Frankincense, Valor, Lavender, Lemon, Harmony, Clarity, Juva Flex, Common Sense and Highest Potential along with a quick reference guide for easy access during stressful times.

Change requires introspection and self-discovery as represented by Percival. Our bodies hold the answer to self-discovery and mastery. One of the easiest way to read the body is through the glandular system which not only controls and regulates the body, but holds the blueprint and destiny for this lifetime. The master gland is the pituitary whose function is to direct the thyroid, commonly associated with metabolism, and the adrenal glands, charged with handling the fight or flight, also known as stress, response. The pancreas gland along with associated organs is responsible for digestion. The rest of the body's functions are carried out by appropriate glands, organs and systems. There are 25 distinct body types each under the direction of its dominant gland, organ or system. Each one has characteristic traits as described earlier in "Points of Connection."

While we operate from all traits, we have two that we express easily or naturally and two that we spend our lives developing. The easiest way to develop recessive traits is to be around people whose dominant traits are the opposite of ours. The down side of being around people who are opposite you, is that they don't think like you think. This gives rise to conflict until both parties have developed their recessive traits enough to appreciate them as strengths when expressed by the other person.

There are many ways to determine your dominant traits. Astrology divides the signs into four elements, color consultants into four seasons, native cultures into four directions, and psychology into four traits. Each of the four elements represents one of the steps necessary for conflict resolution. The following chart reflects the elements and their corresponding frequencies.

TRAITS	ELEMENTS	COMMUNICATION	DIRECTION	SEASON
Emotional	Fire	Dialogue	West	Fall
Physical	Earth	Facts	North	Winter
Mental	Air	Questions	East	Spring
Spiritual	Water	Debate	South	Summer

Identifying your dominant element will go a long way in understanding your communication style as well as your area or areas of weakness. To determine your dominant element, circle the two traits of your body type. In the case of Thyroid, it is mental and spiritual. Identify your dominant element or elements astrologically; Scorpio is water. Look at your communication style and circle what you find yourself doing most often with yourself and others. In my case it is debate. Direction relates to the location of the country where you are most comfortable. For me, living in San Diego, CA, it is south. What is your favorite season? Mine is summer, which is also my season color. My coloring style is soft, subtle, flowing and relaxed, which is a water element that happens to correspond to summer.

The majority of my answers are in the water, debate line which means ultimately finding an answer that is just and fair for both parties. Injustice is the fear stored in the thyroid gland which corresponds to my body type and is one of my core emotional issues or life lessons. Part of my destiny or life mission is to come to a point of resolution by accepting the truth. Knowing truth requires questioning which leads to self purification. The quest for self-realization motivates me to express my passion of doing something worthwhile and making a valuable contribution, which results in my ultimate sense of fulfillment. Likewise, the key to unlocking your destiny is in your body type profile.

AURICULAR THERAPY

Another way to identify emotional patterns is to locate sensitive points on the ears and then refer to the Emotional Reference section. The emotional points on the ears are easily accessible. This is good for an initial release or a quick pickup. As a general clearing use RELEASE on all points. HARMONY is good for a general massage. It is best to begin all therapies by balancing the electrical system of the body with VALOR on the feet (six drops on the bottom of each foot and hold right hand to right foot and left hand to left foot until pulses are in sync). When the electrical system is balanced, the body easily accepts the higher frequency of the emotional oils. You may also wish to use the following oils for specific points. The oils of HARMONY or FORGIVENESS have a positive effect on all points. The points that most need attention will often be tender.

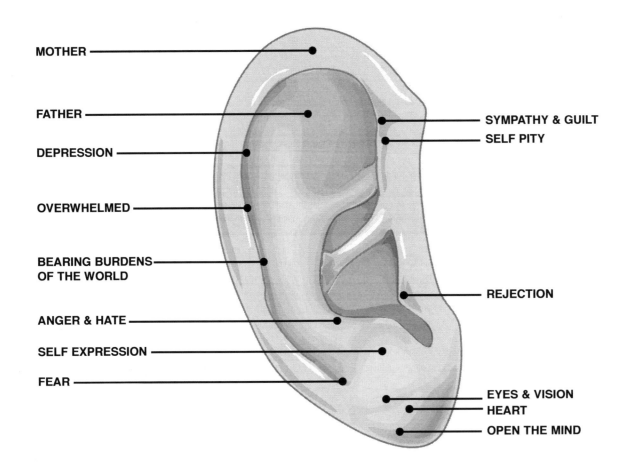

It is not necessary to use all the oils suggested. In fact, that may be overwhelming. Instead, pick an issue or two and use a few oils daily as a continuing support. You can also stimulate the points you are working with by using your fingers, even without oils, several times daily. This is especially useful if depression is an issue. To layer means to immediately apply one oil directly on top of another.

---

[11] Graphic from *Reference Guide for Essential Oils*, by Connie and Alan Higley

MOTHER or FEMALE ISSUES: GERANIUM
Layer YLANG YLANG for sexual abuse issues. Layer with FORGIVENESS and ACCEPTANCE for issues of abandonment. SARA or INNER CHILD may also be very helpful.

FATHER or MALE ISSUES: LAVENDER
Layer with SARA, YLANG YLANG and RELEASE for sexual abuse issues. Layer with HELICHRYSUM for other male abuse issues. HELICHRYSUM helps release deep-seated anger. If related to childhood, GENTLE BABY or INNER CHILD might be very helpful.

DEPRESSION: Most oils help with depression.
Some of the best are HOPE, VALOR, JOY, LAVENDER, WHITE ANGELICA, GENTLE BABY, INNER CHILD, SARA, PEACE & CALMING, CITRUS FRESH, HUMILITY and CHRISTMAS SPIRIT.

OVERWHELMED: Layer ACCEPTANCE and HOPE , VALOR, or GROUNDING.

BEARING THE BURDENS OF THE WORLD: ACCEPTANCE, VALOR and/or RELEASE.
Remember to layer if you are using more than one blend.

ANGER and HATE: FORGIVENESS, ACCEPTANCE, HUMILITY, RELEASE or JOY. Deep-seated anger may also need HELICHRYSUM and/or VALOR to have the strength to forgive. (Layer if using more than one blend.)

SELF-EXPRESSION: MOTIVATION and VALOR for courage to speak out. RELEASE, then ACCEPTANCE or GATHERING for focused expression. INNER CHILD if you have lost your identity. SURRENDER for excessive expression. JOY to enjoy life to the fullest.

FEAR: This point is almost always tender when fear is present. VALOR layered with ACCEPTANCE, HARMONY, RELEASE, or JOY. SARA, INNER CHILD or GENTLE BABY if related to childhood. INTO THE FUTURE for fear of the future.

OPEN THE MIND: 3 WISE MEN associated with the crown and navel. ACCEPTANCE, FRANKINCENSE, GATHERING, CLARITY, MOTIVATION, SANDALWOOD, MAGNIFY YOUR PURPOSE , RELEASE.

HEART: JOY, FORGIVENESS, and ACCEPTANCE for self acceptance. BERGAMOT for grief. SARA for abuse. GENTLE BABY, INNER CHILD if associated with childhood issues. AROMA LIFE will help strengthen the heart and lower blood pressure.

EYES and VISION (inner or outer): INTO THE FUTURE, DREAM CATCHER, ACCEPTANCE, 3 WISE MEN, and/or ENVISION for vision of goals. To improve eyesight: 10 drops LEMONGRASS, 5 CYPRESS, 3 EUCALYPTUS in 1/2 oz. of V6 mixing oil.

REJECTION: ACCEPTANCE layered with FORGIVENESS. If there was rejection from the mother, add GERANIUM. If from the father, LAVENDER.

SELF–PITY: JOY, ACCEPTANCE, and FORGIVENESS. PANAWAY if very painful, may be felt as heaviness in chest. RELEASE, then VALOR to find the courage to move beyond the feeling.

SYMPATHY & GUILT: JOY, INSPIRATION, RELEASE, PANAWAY, ACCEPTANCE. Generally felt more in the neck and head. We need to be compassionate with others, not sympathetic. Sympathy is simply feeling the feelings along with them. To be compassionate is to understand and offer a helping hand.

WRITING TECHNIQUES

While there are a number of different ways to release buried emotions, one of the most effective is writing. Writing incorporates visual, auditory (inner voice), and kinesthetic senses. Writing connects the emotions (heart) with the expression (hand/physical) as the nerve branch that supplies the heart also supplies the hand. Since writing provides a forum for the unconscious to speak, it is essential to allow whatever comes up to be expressed uncensored.

Mother/Father Issues

Our first experience with people is our experience with our parents or guardians. Consequently, our opinions, beliefs, and expectations about women are based on our experiences with Mom, and those about men from Dad. One of the first steps in personal growth is to release buried emotions around parents or major authority figures in our lives.

A simple, yet profound, method of letting go of the past is to take a large notebook and start writing. Begin with the parent or person you had the greatest difficulty with when you were growing up and write down everything you would have liked to have said but felt you couldn't. As you write, feelings will randomly surface from different time periods in your life. When you run out of something to write or feel blocked, ask yourself, "and".... then the next wave will surface. Initially, everything that comes up will be negative. Then it will shift and you will begin to understand where the person was coming from. As you continue to write, your attitude will shift toward compassion for them. Next, you will begin to see what you learned from your experiences and the gifts you have received. Continue writing on the positive side as long as you like[12]..

Once you have completed writing everything you would have liked to say, which may fill several notebooks, you will notice your relationship with this person will change. The common thought is that the other person changed, when in reality it is you.

Taking Personal Responsibility

Having cleared basic mother/father issues, it is time to take responsibility for what you are creating in your own life. There are five elements that create your experience, and they can be addressed in a five part writing program[13]. For this section, you'll need 5 notebooks or one large notebook with 5 sections or divisions. Use one book or division for one of each of the following 5 sections:

1. Negative—feelings and thoughts

2. Positive—feelings and thoughts

3. Goals—in 10 years

4. Desires

5. Blueprint—how you structure your life to make your desires and goals manifest

Start by writing in the Negative book, as this allows you to clear unresolved issues and release the feelings. Since most of us have buried emotions for years, there is a lot to release—more than can be done in one day—so you may want to set aside a definite period of time to write on a regular basis.

---

[12] *Velvet Hammer*, Lee Gibson, Ph.D. PEAKE Seminar
[13] Gary Young. N.D. Phoenix Training Seminar. 1999

Finish each session by writing at least one positive statement in the Positive, Goals, or Desires book, as this builds self-esteem.

Writing is more effective than talking into a tape because it connects with a visual sense. Using a lead pencil helps transfer emotion.

Blind writing is a good way of allowing the unconscious to speak, especially when the conscious mind is strong and likes to control. Simply close your eyes and write. When finished, read it back.

There are specific oils that can help you clear and release as you do the writing program:

SURRENDER—releases negative thoughts. Either diffuse through the air, place on temples and/or smell the oil.

GATHERING—helps if your mind jumps from one subject to another, or thoughts become scattered. If you tend to be overanalytical, swipe across your forehead starting from your left temple using 2-3 fingers on your right hand, and breathe deeply. This will switch you from your left to right brain. If you have trouble being focused or difficulty accepting yourself, reverse the motion using 2-3 fingers on your left hand and swipe across your forehead starting from your right temple, and breathe deeply. GATHERING helps you release your emotions and feelings.

ACCEPTANCE—difficulty accepting emotion. Apply over the 3rd eye (located at the center of your forehead) before you lose it with excessive, uncontrollable emotion.

FORGIVENESS—anything for which you feel guilty. Say, "It's okay," and apply clockwise on the navel several times.

HOPE—feeling depressed or despair. Rub on top of ears or rim of ear.

BRAIN POWER or CLARITY—for brain fog. Apply on temples or under nose.

JOY—enhances feelings of self-esteem. Place on heart, especially when ready to complete writing session.

WHITE ANGELICA—protection from bombardment. Helps you to maintain a positive space. Apply to sternum, shoulders, and nape of neck. Always end with WHITE ANGELICA because as you clear, you become more sensitive to energies around you and you want to be selective of the energy frequencies you hold in your energy field.

Dr. D. Gary Young successfully used this writing technique in treating chronic degenerative diseases like multiple sclerosis, cancer, arthritis and lupus. Stuffed negative emotions and thoughts lead to explosions either as emotional outbursts or internally in the form of disease. Dwelling on negative thoughts and feelings magnifies them. The way out is to process or understand the lesson, forgive yourself for needing to learn the lesson, forgive others for having brought the lesson to you, and release the blocked emotion by allowing it to move to its opposite polarity—choosing how you would like to respond in future situations—and release the pattern from your cellular memory.

Once you clear the major issues in your life, the more subtle ones surface. Major issues are directly related to your thoughts and are like bacteria in that they can be devastating and even fatal. Subtle issues are associated with old thought residue and are like viruses in the way they drain your energy and cause fatigue. Funguses and yeasts are insidious and associated with beliefs held by family and society, commonly known as race consciousness. The first step is to clean up your own thoughts, or take dominion over your own household. This is what it means to be responsible. Your thoughts are ultimately the only area you can control, and it's your thoughts that determine your reality.

According to Dr. Young, keeping busy prevents negative space, and an idle mind leads to negative emotion. This occurs because an idle mind is receptive and will attract whatever is around it. The mind is like a radio, tuning in and playing the strongest frequency. To stop the mind chatter, provide a positive thought like an affirmation and listen to positive tapes and music. Working on a challenging or worthwhile project allows your mind to be creative. A creative mind channels energy in a positive manner, making it easy to maintain a positive space.

Now that you have done your homework, you get to express your talents. This is a time of self-discovery, looking within to find your passion and avenue of creativity. Everything you need to know is embodied within you. Listen to your body and your inner knowing. Learning your body type validates what you intuitively know and provides a basis to fill in the gaps.

SUPPORTING YOURSELF

Accepting Yourself

Achieving awareness requires that you recognize what is "you" and accept yourself. A helpful exercise is to stand in front of a mirror and look yourself in the eyes. Maintain eye contact while you say with conviction and sincerity 100 times: "I accept you as you are." (You can set a timer rather than keeping count if you wish). Once you have accepted yourself and your present reality, you can begin to change it.

Changing Beliefs

Changing a limiting belief requires being conscious of it and choosing a new direction. All of our emotions can be divided into two categories: *Love* and *Fear*. Anything that is negative, restrictive, or limiting is fear-based. That which is positive, compassionate, and supportive is love-based. Changing the old thought pattern requires changing the words or direction we give our subconscious. One very important step toward shifting consciousness is to eliminate limiting words from our vocabulary. Two of the most commonly used words are *Can't* and *Try*.

Can't translates to won't or will not. It also relates to being helpless rather than being self-responsible. If you don't have an immediate answer for something, you can use statements such as "I choose to know," "It will come to me," or "I'll find out."

The word *Try* means to attempt to do or accomplish. Attempt means to make an effort at, effort extended toward, but not accomplishing or succeeding. Try relates to being stuck or sitting on the fence.

Succeeding, achieving, or accomplishing a goal requires seeing it done. Rather than saying you will "try" to do something, make a commitment either to do it or not and allow your words to reflect your decision. Doing so will eliminate wasted effort as well as misunderstandings and hurt feelings in relationships. If you are not sure you can commit to something, say so with comments such as, "I will consider it," or "At this point, I will plan on it."

Changing your reality requires honest communication between your conscious and subconscious mind. Your subconscious takes everything it receives literally; it is like a huge database and reflects back that which is put in.

Taking charge of your life requires having a direction or goals that make you conscious of where you are going. What holds people back is the fear of the unknown and a certain comfort level with what is known, even if it is painful. It takes energy to change; this is why support groups, inspirational material, and positive friends make such a difference. Ultimately, it takes *Faith* , defined as "face it," meaning facing the fear. *Fear* is false evidence appearing real.

MUSCLE TESTING PROCEDURE
FOR PRACTITIONERS AND THERAPISTS

1. Therapy localization uses a test muscle as an indicator to determine the presence of a disconnection in the energy field. To therapy localize, locate a strong muscle you want to use as an indicator, touch the point in question and retest the muscle. A weakening of the previously strong muscle indicates a positive response. To determine the presence of an emotional pattern, touch the emotional points on the frontal eminences. If the previously strong muscle goes weak, an emotional pattern is present.

2. Identify the emotion by asking the patient what issues or emotions he or she is currently struggling with, and test with the indicator muscle. Once a definite response has been found, confirm it by contacting or "therapy localizing" the emotional points and the corresponding organ alarm point for the identified emotion.

   If the patient is unable to identify an emotion, go to the area of complaint and therapy localize the organ alarm point. Confirm with the emotional points and the emotion.

3. Ask the patient to feel the emotion; then the emotion on the "other side." Testing by using the indicator muscle helps solidify the emotion into the patient's experience. Explain the emotions as necessary for the patient's understanding. State the "way out." Test the indicator muscle and explain as indicated.

4. Have the patient smell the oil, place a drop in your non-dominant hand and rub the oil clockwise to activate. Place the oil on the alarm point, or points if bilateral, and the emotional points. While applying the oil, state the emotion, the "other side" and the "way out," encouraging the patient to connect with his/ her feelings and allow them to surface.

5. Test the patient for frequency of use. Occasionally, one application is enough. Depending on how deepseated the pattern, patients usually need to apply the oil 3, 7, 10 or 18 times per day for 1, 3, or 7 weeks. When working on several emotions, the oils may be layered applying one immediately after another. The oil for each emotion may be applied as close as 15 minutes apart, so patients can use them before and after work when they have a chance to focus on the emotions.

   If the patient is not able to use the oil as frequently as required or needs to interrupt usage, he/she can extend the time period. Frequency and duration of treatment is an indication of the depth of the emotional pattern, not an absolute. Some patients may need to extend treatment, so recheck once they feel complete.

6. Review with the patient what he/she will be doing:
   a) feel the emotion and smell the oil,
   b) apply the oil to the alarm point and connect with the "other side" emotion,
   c) apply the oil to the emotional points and state the "way out."

Talk therapy is essential in understanding the situation, but it takes more than head knowledge to change a pattern. The pattern needs to be released from the body for a conditioned response to change. Once understood, the stored emotions can be released from the cellular memory through the alarm points. Aromatherapy is used to access the seat of the emotion in the limbic system of the brain. Identifying the (negative) emotion, its (positive) complementary "other side," and the lesson with the "way out" of the uncomfortable state brings the lesson to conscious awareness. This knowledge provides the awareness necessary to learn the lesson and change the behavior pattern. Smelling and applying specific essential oils to the areas where the emotions are stored allows the cellular pattern to be released from the body, so the emotional pattern can change.

ENHANCEMENT TECHNIQUES

Using these techniques can enhance the clearing process by facilitating the release of the emotional charge and reducing the number of repetitions necessary to change the pattern.

Fully Experience the Feelings

1. Identify the emotion. Feel the emotion and fully embody the emotion and everything associated with the emotion.

2. Smell the oil, breathing the emotion in and out. On the third breath allow the frequency of the emotion to raise you to the opposite side. (If the initial emotion is anger, stay with anger until it rises to laughter.) To assist in the release of the emotion, breathe in the positive emotion (laughter) and breathe out, releasing the negative (anger).

3. Once you have reached the opposite emotion (laughter), apply the oil *Purification* and say the statement with consciousness (My direction is clear) and keep saying it until the energy releases and clears. This is when you reach a still point and the energy is no longer moving.

When working with a facilitator, the facilitator will hold the space, allowing the client to move into the energy. The key is to hold the space without judgment, so the client can fully feel the emotion. For maximum effectiveness, it is best that the facilitator be cleared of the emotional pattern prior to working with the client.

Clear While You Sleep

Program your subconconscious to work on emotions while you sleep. Diffuse the essential oil by setting the travel diffuser by your bed with the oil for the emotion you are clearing.

Smell the oil and connect with the emotion. Apply the oil to the alarm points and feel the opposite emotion. Touch the emotional points on your forehead and say the statement. You may work on several emotions simultaneously.

Muscle Testing

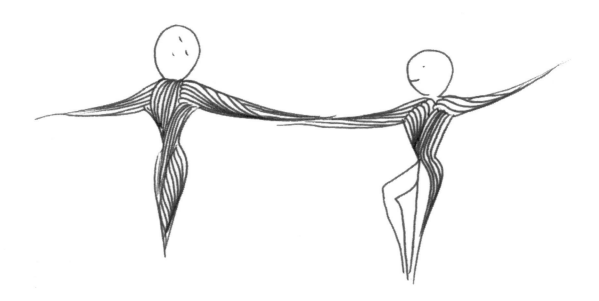

THE BENEFITS OF MUSCLE TESTING

Muscle testing is a simple technique that allows you to communicate directly with your body. It can tell you exactly what your body needs at any given moment. I have found it to be by far, the most valuable tool I have ever used. It was through muscle testing that I was able to determine which oils were associated with which emotion.

Muscle testing is really very simple. It's just a way of communicating with your subconscious. This is important because it's your subconscious that is in charge of running and maintaining your body.

To test something, all you need to do is to find a strong indicator muscle and check its ability to remain strong in relationship to different stimuli. These will be the different oils you are considering using, where to use them, and how often.

INTERPRETING THE RESULTS

The muscles most commonly used in this procedure are the shoulder muscles, the chest and arm muscles, or the back muscles. When tested, if the muscles stay firm under the pressure that is applied, the substance being assessed has a positive or beneficial effect on your body. If the pressure causes the muscle to weaken or "give", then the substance tested has a negative effect and will use more energy to be processed or eliminated than it provides.

When a muscle tests weak, it may be demonstrated in varying degrees. Weakness may be dramatic, indicating a definite "No" for that substance, or moderately weak or "spongy".

"Sponginess" suggests that the substance is not particularly beneficial to your system, nor is it detrimental.

THE ORIGIN AND BASIS OF MUSCLE TESTING

In 1964, Dr. George Goodheart, a Chiropractic Physician, discovered that he could derive information about the body through a process of testing muscles. He found a way to bypass the conscious filter of the mind so he could communicate directly with the physical body. This profound discovery opened the door to being able to determine exactly what was going on in the body. It greatly enhanced the physical ability to diagnose, enabling physicians to be more specific. For example, if someone knew they had a urinary tract infection which could be confirmed by a urinalysis, the next question would be "What's causing it?" By using muscle testing and the acupuncture alarm points, physicians could determine whether it was coming from the bladder, urinary tract, or kidneys.

Muscle testing's greatest value is in providing the ability to diagnose physical problems by communicating directly with the body. Through using muscle testing, Dr. Goodheart demonstrated the interrelationship of muscles to internal body functions.

Basis of Muscle Testing

Muscle testing is based on the standard muscle strength tests used to determine muscle disability. These tests were developed by Kendall, Kendall, & Wadsworth, medical authorities on kinesiology, which is the science of human muscular movements (Muscles: Testing and Function, 2nd ed., Baltimore, 1971).

How Muscle Testing Works

Muscle testing works by using the biophysical and mechanical links between muscles, joints, nerves, and organs to identify specific requirements and body imbalances. *The method involves placing a reasonable amount of pressure on a muscle or group of muscles, and determining the individual's ability to resist the pressure.*

Muscle testing is an interesting concept, and how it works can be understood both physically and mentally. From a physical standpoint, we know that the body possesses an energy field that permeates and surrounds it. Muscle testing takes advantage of fluctuations in this bioenergy field. If the energy flow is disturbed or interrupted, the motor nerve impulses are affected, resulting in decreased muscle strength.

Traditional Chinese medicine has mapped the flow of energy in this field as it moves through the body along pathways called meridians. It is along these meridians that the Chi, or life force of the body, flows. The Chinese have demonstrated the effect of this flow on health through the science of acupuncture, which is a diverse system of treatment that can be applied to many ailments.

Using Kirlian photography, this energy field produced by the life force can be seen radiating outward to form an aura around the body. This occurs in all living things—humans, animals, and even the leaves of plants and trees. While this energy field is normally not visible to the naked eye, it can be easily seen in the pictures this type of photography produces.

Why Muscle Testing Works

The mechanics of muscle testing can also be explained in terms of a subconscious mental response. **The subconscious mind that controls the internal bodily functions knows what foods and substances the body needs.** The body is always in perfect alignment with the subconscious, so it always accurately reflects its needs.

Look at the effect that emotions have on the body. Since they are subconsciously generated, they are linked to corresponding physiological changes in the body. Anger, for instance, causes increases in blood pressure, heart rate, respiration, and muscle tension. Other emotions, too, have physical manifestations in the body that are directly related to the subconscious response.

Muscle testing utilizes this harmony between the subconscious mind and the physical body. It allows us to communicate with the subconscious and assess its reaction to stimuli by using the body as both a transmitter and a receiver.

When a substance is placed in contact with the body, the subconscious reacts to it as beneficial, neutral, or harmful. This produces the physical response of either increasing or decreasing muscle strength depending on its effect on the body or the subconscious.

HOW TO MUSCLE TEST

Basic Techniques

Choose the muscle to be used as an indicator. Any muscle or muscle group can be used. When the person being tested is stronger than the person doing the testing, it's best to choose a muscle that can be isolated and tested by itself. This provides a more accurate test because it reduces the likelihood of recruitment from the surrounding muscles. When the person being tested is noticeably weaker than the person doing the testing (man testing woman).using a larger muscle or group of muscles helps to balance relative strength. Since muscle mass is different for men, women, and children, instructions on how to test for several muscle strengths has been provided. Select accordingly. The following suggested techniques (explained later) generally work best:

• Man testing woman—use shoulder muscle.

• Woman testing man—use upper chest, or back muscle.

• Man or woman testing child—use a combination of chest and arm muscles.

• Self-testing—use hand and finger muscles.

Important Points

•*Be objective.* This means making sure you are not holding the thought of your desired outcome in your mind while performing the test. Your subconscious wants to please you so if you really want something and think about it while testing, you can get a wrong answer. Let your mind go into neutral, or focus on accurately performing the test.

• *This is not a strength contest.* A weak muscle response during a test does not indicate a deficiency in the muscle.

The muscle is fine. It only tests weak in response to what is being tested because nerve impulses are being interrupted. The muscle will again test strong once the indicator is removed.

• When working with someone who has not done muscle testing before, go through the range of motion once or twice so they can become familiar with the procedure *Misunderstandings can lead to inaccurate results.*

Pressure Applied

• You will know the muscle is strong when you feel it "lock in" or hold. This usually occurs within the first 15 degrees of the muscle's range of motion. If it doesn't hold, use the other arm or select another muscle.

• A moderate amount of pressure should be smoothly applied to the muscle, and then gradually released.

• Avoid sudden movements and exert no more pressure than necessary to determine muscle strength.

• Do not attempt to overpower the muscle, as this could lead to false results.

• Exert the same amount of pressure on the muscle with each test, noticing the differences in the responses of the muscle in the various tests. If unsure of the muscle reaction, ask the person being tested how it felt, then evaluate the results.

NOTE: You can clarify your results at this time if your response did not seem well-defined by using the Enhancement Technique (Scott Walker, D.C.). Turn your head to the right while the person being tested turns his or her head to the left so that you are both facing the same direction. Muscle testing this way will exaggerate differences in the responses that previously may have been only slight.

Muscle Isolation

Don't recruit: Make sure that the person being tested does not use any additional muscles to strengthen his or her response to the testing. The body wants to be strong and will often use other strong muscles to compensate for weak ones. This is done by slightly changing the position of the arm, bending the elbow, or tilting the body. Since the goal is to isolate a muscle, bringing other muscles into play makes testing more difficult and will often invalidate results.

Specific Tests

The purpose of the following tests is to determine strength or weakness.

• Strength, or a "Yes" response, is present when the muscle is strong and locked. Take care not to overpower the muscle you are testing.

• A "No" response is when the muscle is weak. The easiest way to learn muscle testing is to begin by working with another person, testing each other. Once you feel confident with muscle testing, you are ready to start testing yourself.

TEST 1: Man Testing Woman
Use when a person of larger muscle mass (man) **is testing someone smaller** (woman).

This test uses the deltoid, or shoulder muscle.

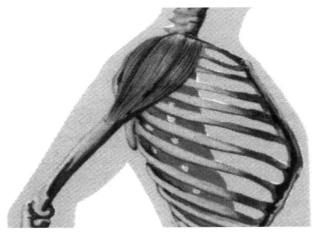

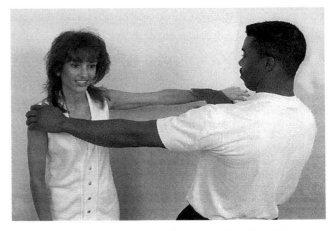

Arm extended straight out to the side.

1. From a sitting or standing position, the woman extends one arm either forward or to the side so that it is horizontal to the floor.

2. The palm of the hand of the woman should be down and elbow straight, but not locked.

3. The muscles of the arm, chest, and back should be as relaxed as possible so as not to reinforce the shoulder with allied muscles.

4. The man stands in front or to the side of the woman and exerts downward pressure on the arm just above the wrist. This determines the strength of the shoulder muscle.

5. If the man is considerably stronger than the woman, the woman may bend the elbow, bringing the hand inward, so the man's leverage will be reduced when pressing at the elbow.

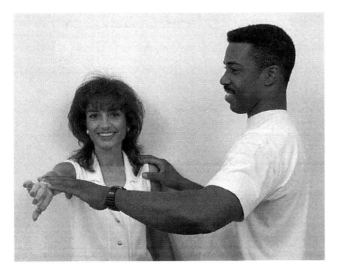

Arm extended straight forward at a right angle to body.

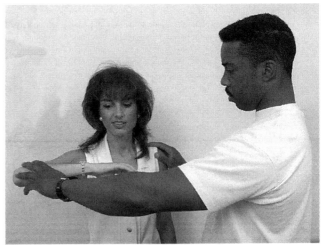

Arm out with elbow bent.
Bending the elbow decreases the leverage, making testing easier for the person being tested.

TEST 2: Woman Testing Man

This test is often useful when the tester (woman) has substantially less muscle mass than the person being tested (man), or when both are about the same size. (This can also be two women or two men of comparable strength). It uses the pectoralis major clavicular or upper portion of the chest muscle that attaches to the clavicle.

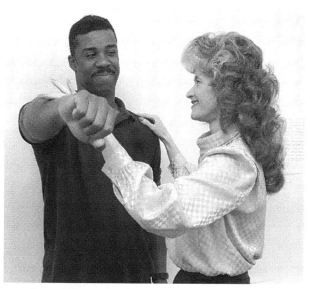

Starting position with a strong or "Yes" response.

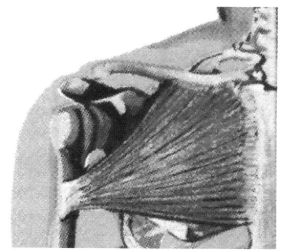

Pectoralis Major Clavicular Muscle

2. Tester then applies pressure on the arm above the wrist, but instead of pushing straight downward, the force is exerted at a 45 degree angle down and away from the body.

1. As in Test #1, the person being tested extends one arm forward with the elbow locked and the palm turned outward with the thumb pointing toward the floor.

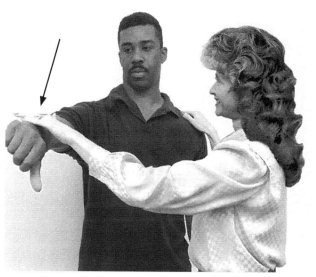

Ending position with a weak or "No" response.

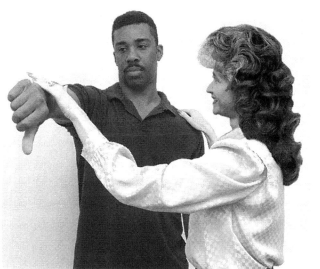

Apply steady pressure at a 45 degree angle away from the body.

TEST 3: Alternative Test

Another test that is easy to use engages the latissimus dorsi, or back muscle. **This may be used when both people are the same size,** or either person is larger. This test can easily be done in either a standing or lying position.

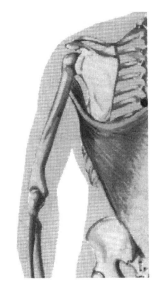

Latissimus Dorsi Muscle

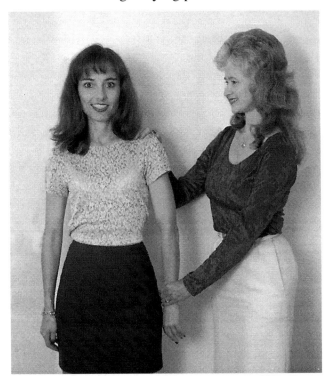

Starting position with a strong or "Yes" response.

1. Have the person being tested stand with one arm extended downward next to her/his side and rotated inward so that the palm of the hand and elbow face outward, away from the body.

2. The tester applies steady pressure just above the wrist of the person being tested, pulling in an outward direction. The other hand is placed on the person's shoulder to stabilize the body.

3. If the muscle is strong and stays close to the body, you have a "Yes" response.

4. Weakness will be apparent within the first 5-15 degrees when the muscle fails to engage or "lock in", moving away from the body.

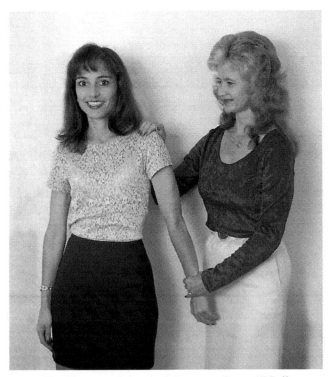

Ending position with a weak or "No" response.

TEST 4: Testing Children (ages 4-8)

In this test, both the chest and arm muscles are used. This exception to the isolation of a single muscle increases the child's resistance to pressure from the adult.

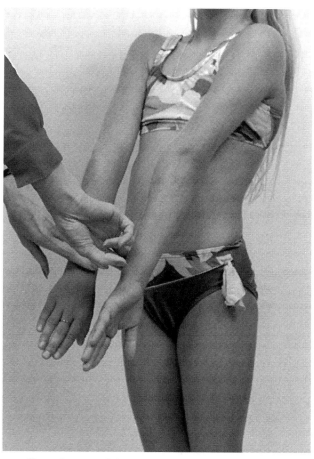

Starting position with a strong or "Yes" response (arms together).

1. Both arms are held straight and extended downward in front of the body, staying close to the body.

2. The palms of the hands are turned outward and the backs of the wrists are held together.

3. The tester, standing in front of the person being tested, tries to separate the wrists by simultaneously applying pressure on each arm above the wrist in an outward direction. When children are small, you need only use your index fingers above the wrists.

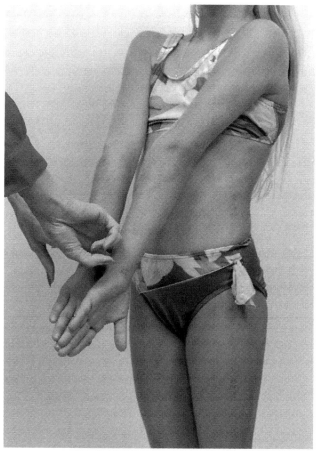

Ending position when test is weak or "No" response (arms apart).

NOTE: When testing young children it is often helpful to tell them to "push your wrists together" since they are generally better able to understand this than the command, "resist" or "keep your arms together."

TEST 5: Testing with Body Movement

The first time your experience this test it is best to have someone present to catch you, because you may have considerable body movement. Some people find this test to be a good one to use for self testing, while others need to have someone present to assist.

1. Take your shoes off, especially if you are wearing high heels. Stand with your feet flat on the floor and relax, allowing your body to move.

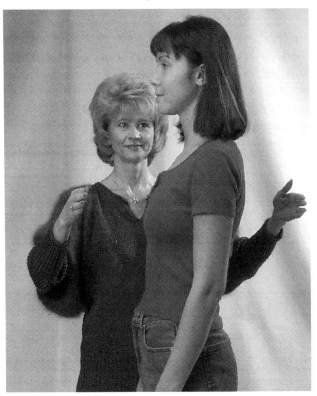

Neutral or starting position

2. Have someone stand, ready to catch you, with their hands on both sides of your body.

3. Close your eyes and relax your body. Say "Yes" deliberately three times and allow your body to move. Have the person standing beside you observe the direction you move and catch you if needed.

4. Close your eyes and relax your body. Say "No" deliberately three times and allow your body to move. Have the person standing beside observe the direction you move and catch you if needed.

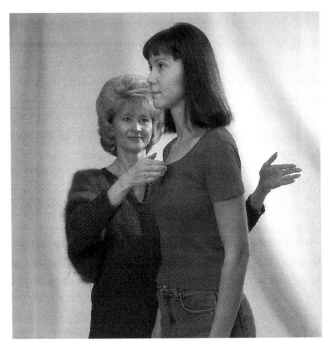

5. Determine the direction your body moves for "Yes" and for "No". Some people move forward for "Yes" and backward for "No"; for others it is the opposite. Some sway clockwise or counterclockwise, while others show little if any movement. If your body moves in a definite direction, this is a simple, accurate test you can use.

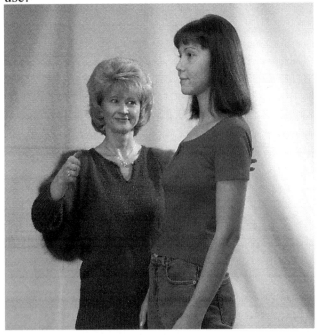

Test 6: Self Testing

In these two simple **methods for testing yourself**, you are opposing your own muscles rather than those of another. Remaining objective, so you will get accurate results, is more difficult in these methods and probably should be used only when you are more experienced at muscle testing.

These tests allow for varying degrees of weakness, as do the tests using the larger muscles. While I have specified use of left and right hands in these directions, reversal of the left hand for the right may also be used.

Self-Testing: "O" Ring Method

1. Touch the tips of the thumb and index finger of your left hand together to form a circular opening ("O" ring).

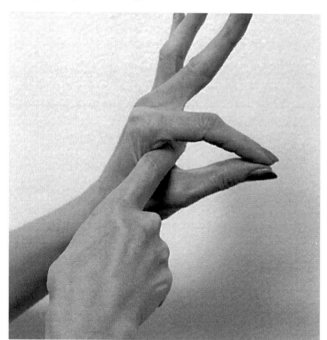

"O" ring with inserted finger

2. Insert the index finger of your right hand into the opening so it rests against your left palm.

3. While continuing to hold thumb and index finger together, quickly and forcefully move your right index finger toward the tips of the left thumb and index finger, attempting to break through the barrier formed by these two fingers.

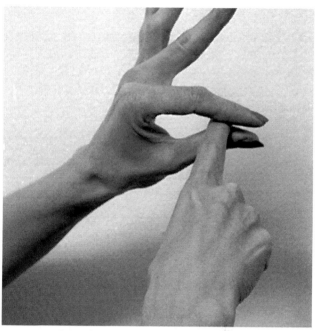

Moving finger against barrier

Begin this movement as far back in the circle as possible to get a "running start" at the barrier.

4. If you don't break through the barrier, the muscle test is strong. Breaking through indicates a weak muscle response. Test results here will be a definite "Yes" (strong) or "No" (weak).

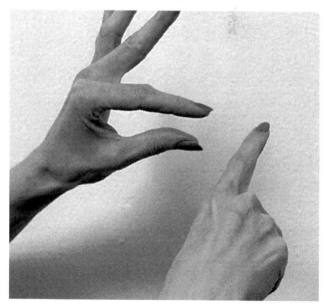

Finger breaks through barrier: "No" response.

Self-Testing: Muscle Resistance Method

1. Touch the thumb and little finger of your left hand together.

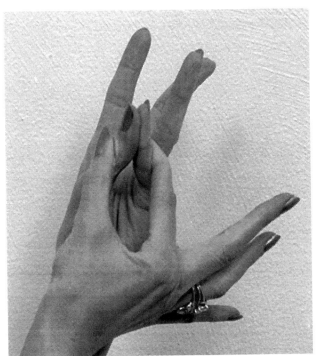

Strong or "Yes" response with no separation

2. Grasp this with the thumb and index finger of your right hand so that pressure is applied, holding your left thumb and little finger together.

3. Try to separate the thumb and little finger of your left hand by exerting pressure against the fingers of your right hand. Inability to separate indicates a "strong response", intermittent (on and off) separation is a "moderate response", and complete separation, a "weak response".

This method allows you to have a "Moderate" response in addition to a definite "Yes" or "No".

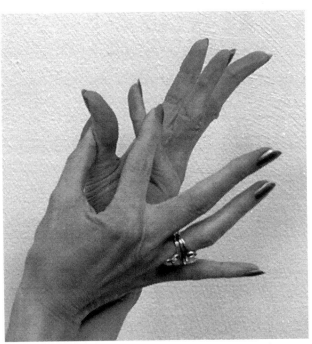

Weak or "No" response with separation

IMPLEMENTING MUSCLE TESTING

Once you have determined the muscle test you want to use, test the muscle itself. This is known as "testing in the clear," and is done for the following reasons:

- To make sure you have a strong muscle.

- To test the relative strength of this muscle to determine how much pressure should be applied.

- To acquaint the person with the test, and establish a "baseline" so you know how a strong muscle feels.

- Following this procedure, you are now ready to evaluate the need for different oils by assessing responses to them.

Method

1. **Place the oil to be tested within the bioenergy field of the person being tested.** The most accurate results are obtained when the person being tested can smell the oil. While this is ideal, it is not mandatory. The person being tested can hold the bottle of oil in a free hand, or simply touch it to the body. When self-testing and both hands are occupied, use your arm to hold the oil against your side or chest, or put it inside your belt against your abdomen.

2. **Perform the test and compare the muscle strength results to that of the "baseline" test.** A strong response indicates a definite "Yes", a spongy response means the substance is helpful but not the most appropriate or best choice, and a weak response means "No, definitely not now".

3. **Once the appropriate oil or oils have been found, determine where it needs to be applied.** This can be done by touching the bottle to the corresponding alarm point, the feet, or any of the general points on the nose if the requirement is to smell it.

The closer the actual substance is to the point (without actually applying it in case of a possible negative response) the more accurate the test results. Touching the point or visualizing and verbally saying the location can also be effective.

HELPFUL HINTS

1. When you begin muscle testing, first test foods or substances that you know are "good" or "bad" for you. This will give you the experience of feeling the responses and allow you to understand what you can expect.

2. If test results seem inconsistent, you could be dehydrated. Drink some water, then test again.

3. Take off your jewelry, watch, and anything else that could interfere with energy flow. This will help ensure the accuracy of your test results.

Accuracy

The purpose of muscle testing is to obtain accurate answers. The key to accuracy in muscle testing is remaining objective. It's usually easier to do this when you are being tested by someone else, but with practice you'll be able to maintain your objectivity while testing yourself. Check your accuracy by testing the foods or substances that you know produce a dramatic "Yes" or "No" response.

Like everything else, proficiency in muscle testing requires practice. Once you become skillful, it will be easy to determine which oils are needed, when and where to apply them and for how long. Eventually you'll find yourself developing an intuitive awareness about what your body needs, and then you'll only test to confirm what you already know.

BIBLIOGRAPHY

Essential Science Publishing, Compiled by, DR *Peoples's Desk Reference for Essential Oils*, Salem, UT, Essential Science Publishing, (1999)

Farmer, Kathy, *Unlocking Emotions with Essential Oils*

Friedmann, Terry, M.D. *Freedom Through Health*, North Glenn, CO, Harvest Publishers (1998)

Herzog, Roberta, D.D. *The Akashic Reading Guidelines*, P.O. Box 448, Scotland Neck, NC, Roberta Herzog Publisher (1993) 252-826-0837 www.robertaherzog

Higley, Connie and Alan, *Reference Guide for Essential Oils*, Orem, UT, Abundant Health (1998)

Mein, Carolyn, D.C., *Different Bodies, Different Diets*, San Diego, CA, Vision Ware Press (1998)

Mein, Carolyn, D.C., *Different Bodies, Different Diets*, New York City, NY, HarperCollins Publishers Inc. (2001)

Myss, Caroline, Ph.D., *Why People Don't Heal And How They Can*, New York City, NY, Harmony Books (1997)

Pearsall, Paul P., *The Heart Code*, New York City, NY, Broadway Books (1998)

Pert, Candace B., Ph.D., *Molecules of Emotion:Why You Feel the Way You Feel*, New York City, NY, Scribner (1997)

Page, Ken, *The Way It Works*, Bastrop, TX, Clearlight Arts (1997)

Truman, Carol, *Feelings Buried Alive Never Die*, St. George, UT, Olympus Distributing Corporation (1991)

Ulfelder, Susan, N.D., Personal Communication, Bethesda, MD

Young, Gary, N.D., *Aromatherapy: The Essential Beginning*, Salt Lake City, UT, Essential Press Publishing (1996)

RESOURCES

Different Bodies, Different Diets
This book solves the "one diet fits all" mystery with the 25 Body Type System. The system is based on the premise that every person has a dominant gland, organ or system that is present at birth and remains dominant throughtout one's life. This dominant gland is what determines certain physical characteristics, psychological and emotional traits.

Fitness-Fun-Ball™
The easiest way to exercise is with the Fitness-Fun™. Ball Incorporate exercise into your lifestyle by using a Fitness-Fun-Ball™ as a chair. The weakest point of the body is the pelvis which results in weakness of the lower abdominal muscles and low back pain. Sitting on the ball forces you to use your pelvic and lower abdominal muscles. This improves posture, reduces wrist problems, and stimulates cerebral-spinal fluid movement, resulting in increased alertness and mental clarity.

Core Fitness DVD
Focuses on effectively strengthening the abdominal muscles with the Pilates-based exercises using the Fitness Ball.

Tara Diamond, MS, BMS, is a spiritual healer and counselor, human design analyst, artist and teacher. Her 20 years of transpersonal healing experiences have developed into a deeply intuitive healing technique. She was a minister with The Teaching of the Inner Christ, and for 10 years taught astral healing, prayer therapy, and inner sensitivity training. Currently, she works with individuals, clearing the energy field of astral influences that affect their psycho-spiritual development.
Tara Diamond: (619) 888-9237, www.taradiamond.com

Young Living Essential Oils™
Dedicated to restoring a healing message and knowledge to the people of the world, Young Living Essential Oils™ is committed to supplying the highest grade of essential oils. To ensure purity and quality, Young Living raises, harvests, and distills many of their essential oils. Founded by Dr. Gary Young, N.D., Young Living Essential Oils™ are distributed through personal representatives. Or may be ordered directly by calling 800-371-2928, #10586.

Another source of high-quality essential oils is *Original Swiss Aromatics,* P.O. Box 6842, San Rafael, CA 94903.

Additional Information:

- **Carolyn L. Mein, D.C. (858) 756-3704**
- *Visit* **our web site: www.bodytype.com**
- *Contact* **your local essential oils distributor**

APPENDIX
Oil Blends by Young Living Essential Oils™

ABUNDANCE™: Orange, Frankincense, Patchouly, Clove, Ginger, Myrrh, Cinnamon Bark, Spruce

ACCEPTANCE™: Rosewood, Geranium, Frankincense, Blue Tansy, Sandalwood, Neroli, in a base of Almond Oil

AROMA LIFE™: Cypress, Marjoram, Helichrysum, Ylang Ylang, in a base of Sesame Seed Oil

AROMA SIEZ™: Basil, Marjoram, Lavender, Peppermint, Cypress

AUSTRALIAN BLUE™: Blue Cypress, Ylang Ylang, Cedarwood, Blue Tansy, White Fir

AWAKEN™: **Joy Essential Blend:** Bergamot, Ylang Ylang, Geranium, Rosewood, Lemon, Mandarin, Jasmine, Roman Chamomile, Palmarosa; **Forgiveness Essential Blend:** Geranium, Rosewood, Melissa, Lemon, Frankincense, Jasmine, Roman Chamomile, Bergamot, Ylang Ylang, Palmarosa, Sandalwood, Angelica, Lavender, Helichrysum, Rose, in a base of Sesame Seed oil; **Present Time Essential Blend:** Neroli, Spruce, Ylang Ylang, in a base of Almond Oil; **Dream Catcher Essential Blend:** Sandalwood, Tangerine, Ylang Ylang, Black Pepper, Bergamot, Juniper, Anisum, Blue Tansy; **Harmony Essential Blend:** Lavender, Sandalwood, Ylang Ylang, Frankincense, Orange, Angelica, Geranium, Spruce, Hyssop, Sage, Lavender, Rosewood, Jasmine, Roman Chamomile, Bergamot, Palmarosa, Rose, in a base of Almond Oil

BELIEVE™: Idaho Balsam Fir, Rosewood, Frankincense

BRAIN POWER™: Sandalwood, Cedarwood, Frankincense, Melissa, Blue Cypress, Lavender, Helichrysum

CHIVALRY™: **Valor Essential Blend:** Spruce, Rosewood, Blue Tansy, Frankincense, in a base of Almond Oil; **Joy Essential Blend:** Bergamot, Ylang Ylang, Geranium, Rosewood, Lemon, Mandarin, Jasmine, Roman Chamomile, Palmarosa, Rose; **Harmony Essential Blend:** Lavender, Sandalwood, Ylang Ylang, Frankincense, Orange, Angelica, Geranium, Spruce, Hyssop, Sage Lavender, Rosewood, Jasmine, Roman Chamomile, Bergamot, Palmarosa, Rose, in a base of Almond Oil; **Gratitude Essential Blend:** Idaho Balsam Fir, Frankincense, Rosewood, Myrrh, Galbanum, Ylang Ylang

CITRUS FRESH™: Orange, Grapefruit, Mandarin, Tangerine, Lemon, Spearmint

CLARITY™: Basil, Cardamom, Rosemary, Peppermint, Rosewood, Geranium, Lemon, Jasmine, Roman Chamomile, Bergamot, Ylang Ylang, Palmarosa

COMMON SENSE™: Frankincense (Boswellia Carteri), Ylang Ylang, Ocotea, Rue, Dorado Azuil, Lime

DI-GIZE™: Tarragon, Ginger, Peppermint, Juniper, Fennel, Lemongrass, Anise, Patchouli

DREAM CATCHER™: Sandalwood, Tangerine, Ylang Ylang, Black Pepper, Bergamot, Juniper, Anise, Blue Tansy

EGYPTIAN GOLD™: Frankincense, Balsam Canada, Lavender, Myrrh, Hyssop, Northern Lights Black Spruce, Cedarwood, Vetiver, Rose, Cinnamon Bark

APPENDIX *of Oil Blends by Young Living Essential Oils*™

ENDO FLEX™: Spearmint, Sage, Geranium, Myrtle, German Chamomile, Nutmeg, in a base of Sesame Seed Oil

EN-R-GEE™: Rosemary, Juniper, Lemongrass, Nutmeg, Idaho Balsam Fir, Clove, Black Pepper

ENVISION™: Spruce, Geranium, Orange, Lavender, Sage, Rose

EXODUS II™: Cassia, Myrrh, Cinnamon Bark, Calamus, Galbanum, Hyssop, Spikenard, Frankincense, in a base of Olive Oil

FORGIVENESS™: Melissa, Geranium, Frankincense, Rosewood, Sandalwood, Angelica, Lavender Lemon, Jasmine, Roman Chamomile, Bergamot, Ylang Ylang, Palmarosa, Helichrysum, Rose, in a base of Sesame Seed Oil

GATHERING™: Lavender, Geranium, Galbanum, Frankincense, Sandalwood, Ylang Ylang, Spruce, Rose, Cinnamon Bark

GENEYUS™: Sacred Frankincense, Blue Cypress, Cedarwood, Idaho Blue Spruce, Palo Santo, Melissa, Northern Lights Black Spruce, Sweet Almond, Bergamot, Myrrh, Vetiver, Geranium, Royal Hawaiian Sandalwood™, Ylang Ylang, Hyssop, Coriander, Rose

GRATITUDE™: Idaho Balsam Fir, Frankincense, Rosewood, Myrrh, Galbanum, Ylang Ylang

GROUNDING™: White Fir, Spruce, Ylang Ylang, Pine, Cedarwood, Angelica, Juniper

HARMONY™: Lavender, Sandalwood, Ylang Ylang, Frankincense, Orange, Angelica, Geranium, Spruce, Hyssop, Sage, Lavender, Rosewood, Jasmine, Roman Chamomile, Bergamot, Palmarosa, Rose

HIGHEST POTENTIAL™: **Australian Blue:** Blue Cypress, Ylang Ylang, Cedarwood, Blue Tansy, White Fir; **Gathering:** Lavender, Geranium, Galbanum, Frankincense, Sandalwood, Ylang Ylang, Spruce, Rose, Cinnamon Bark, Jasmine

HOPE™: Melissa, Juniper, Myrrh, Spruce, in a base of Almond Oil

HUMILITY™: Rosewood, Ylang Ylang, Geranium, Melissa, Frankincense, Spikenard, Myrrh, Neroli, Rose, in a base of Sesame Seed Oil

IMMUPOWER™: Hyssop, Mountain Savory, Cistus, Ravensara, Frankincense, Oregano, Clove, Cumin, Idaho Tansy

INNER CHILD™: Orange, Tangerine, Ylang Ylang, Jasmine, Sandalwood, Lemongrass, Spruce, Neroli

INSPIRATION™: Cedarwood, Spruce, Rosewood, Myrtle, Sandalwood, Frankincense, Mugwort

INTO THE FUTURE™: Clary Sage, Ylang Ylang, White Fir, Idaho Tansy, Frankincense, Jasmine, White Lotus, Juniper, Orange, Cedarwood, in a base of Almond Oil

JOY™: Bergamot, Ylang Ylang, Geranium, Rosewood, Lemon, Mandarin, Jasmine, Roman Chamomile, Palmarosa, Rose

APPENDIX *of Oil Blends by Young Living Essential Oils™*

JUVAFLEX™: Fennel, Geranium, Rosemary, Roman Chamomile, Blue Tansy, Helichrysum, in a base of Sesame Seed Oil

LEGACY™: Angelica, Balsam Fir, Basil, Bay Laurel, Bergamot, Black Pepper, Blue Tansy, Cajeput, Canadian Fleabane, Canadian Red Cedar, Cardamom, Carrot Seed, Cedarwood, Cinnamon Bark, Cistus, Citronella, Clary Sage, Clove, Coriander, Cumin, Cypress, Dill, Douglas Fir, Elemi, Eucalyptus Citriodora, Eucalyptus Dives, Eucalyptus Globulus, Eucalyptus Polybractea, Eucalyptus Radiata, Fennel, Frankincense, Galbanum, Geranium, German Chamomile, Ginger, Goldenrod, Grapefruit, Helichrysum, Hemlock, Hyssop, Idaho Tansy, Jasmine, Juniper, Lavender, Ledum, Lemon, Lemongrass, Lime, Mandarin, Melaleuca Alternifolia, Melaleuca Ericifolia, Melissa, Mountain Savory, Myrrh, Myrtle, Neroli, Nutmeg, Orange, Oregano, Palmarosa, Patchouly, Peppermint, Petitgrain, Pine, Ravensara, Red Fir, Roman Chamomile, Rose, Rose Hip, Rosemary, Rosewood, Sage, Sandalwood, Spearmint, Spikenard, Spruce, Tangerine, Tarragon, Thyme, Valerian,Vetiver, White Fir, Wintergreen, Yarrow, Yellow Pine, Ylang Ylang

LIVE WITH PASSION™: Clary Sage, Ginger, Sandalwood, Jasmine, Angelica, Cedarwood, Melissa, Helichrysum, Patchouli, Neroli

LONGEVITY™: Thyme, Orange, Clove, Frankincense

MAGNIFY YOUR PURPOSE™: Sandalwood, Rosewood, Sage, Nutmeg, Patchouli, Cinnamon Bark, Ginger

MELROSE™: Rosemary, Melaleuca Alternifolia, Clove, Melaleuca Quinquenervia

MOTIVATION™: Roman Chamomile, Ylang Ylang, Spruce, Lavender

PANAWAY™: Wintergreen, Helichrysum, Clove, Peppermint

PEACE & CALMING™: Tangerine, Orange, Ylang Ylang, Patchouli, Blue Tansy

PRESENT TIME™: Neroli, Spruce, Ylang Ylang, in a base of Almond Oil

PURIFICATION™: Citronella, Lemongrass, Rosemary, Melaleuca, Lavendin, Myrtle

R.C.™: Myrtle, Eucalyptus Globulus, Eucalyptus Australiana, Pine, Marjoram, Eucalyptus Citriodora, Lavender, Cypress, Spruce, Eucalyptus Radiata, Peppermint

RELEASE™: Ylang Ylang, Lavandin, Geranium, Sandalwood, Blue Tansy, in a base of Olive Oil

RELIEVE IT™: Spruce, Black Pepper, Hyssop, Peppermint

RUTAVALA™: Lavender, Valerian, Ruta Graveolens

SACRED MOUNTAIN™: Spruce, Ylang Ylang, Idaho Balsam Fir, Cedarwood

SARA™: Ylang Ylang, Geranium, Lavender, Orange, Blue Tansy, Cedarwood, Rose, White Lotus, in a base of Almond Oil

APPENDIX *of Oil Blends by Young Living Essential Oils*™

SURRENDER™: Lavender, Lemon, Roman Chamomile, Spruce, Angelica, German Chamomile

THIEVES™: Clove, Lemon, Cinnamon Bark, Eucalyptus Radiata, Rosemary

3 WISE MEN™: Sandalwood, Juniper, Frankincense, Spruce, Myrrh, in a base of Almond Oil

TRANSFORMATION™: Lemon, Frankincense, Peppermint, Idaho Balsam Fir, Sandalwood, Rosemary, Clary Sage, Cardomom

TRAUMA LIFE™: Frankincense, Sandalwood, Valerian, Lavender, Davana, Spruce, Geranium, Helichrysum, Citrus Hystrix, Rose

VALOR™: Spruce, Rosewood, Blue Tansy, Frankincense, in a base of Almond Oil

WHITE ANGELICA™: Bergamot, Geranium, Myrrh, Sandalwood, Rosewood, Ylang Ylang, Spruce, Hyssop, Melissa, Rose, in a base of Almond Oil

EXERCISE WHILE YOU ARE SITTING!

**Eliminate low back pain and strengthen your abdominals while sitting on the Fitness-Fun-Ball™.
Different body types require different abdominal exercises.**

- Reduce and prevent lower back pain
- Tone your upper and lower abs
- Improve your posture
- Exercise while watching TV
- Noticeable results in 5 minutes a day

*The Core Fitness DVD is based on years of
chiropractic research and Pilates-based exercises*

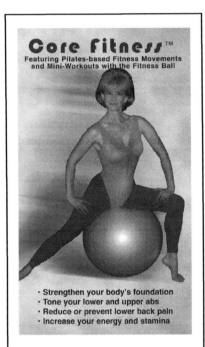

Core Fitness DVD contains:

- 40 minute full body workout.
- Exercises while sitting at your desk.
- 5-10 minute mini workout that targets your weakest areas.

THE IDEAL CHAIR!

**Whether you are doing massage or
sitting at your computer**

- Keeps users more alert and attentive
- Increases energy and creativity
- Enhances functional movement, muscle tone and flexibility
- Increases mobility, stability, balance and postural strength
- Slows the degeneration of the musculoskeletal system
- Reduces stress, tension, headaches and back pain

**Core Fitness DVD $24.95
DVD w/ball purchase $19.95
Fitness Ball Sizes:
55cm - 4'8" to 5'3" $24.95
65cm – 5'3" to 6'0" $29.95
75cm – 6'1" to 6'7" $34.95
Plus Shipping**

**Core Fitness DVD™ & Fitness-Fun-Ball™
Phone: (858) 756-3704 • Fax: (858) 756-6933**

**Carolyn L. Mein, D.C. P.O. Box 8112 Rancho Santa Fe, CA 92067
http://www.bodytype.com**

Rise To Your Highest Potential
By Knowing Your Body Type

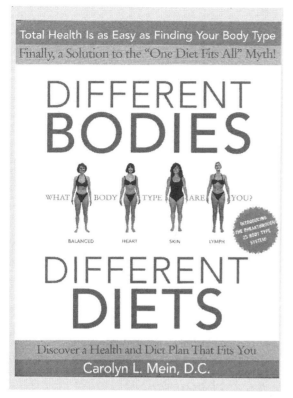

Includes pictures and descripions of each type for
both men and women
Hardcover $27.95

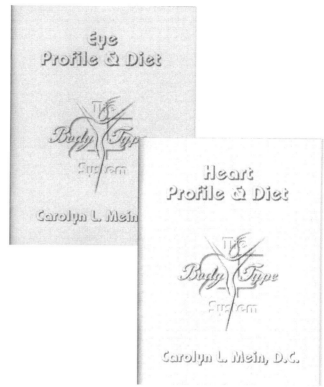

Profile for each individual body type
includes 20-50 menu suggestions for each
type plus 1 week sample menu.
$14.95

· We don't all think alike
· We have different strengths
· We are not motivated by the same things

What would your life be like if you knew your particular strengths, your realistic potential,
where you excel, what motivates you and those around you?

*Rarely are family members the same body type. There are 25 different body types,
each with it's own personality traits and dietary requirements.
Characteristic personality traits may be expressed "at worst" and "at best."
Knowing enhances relationships*

To learn more about *The 25 Body Type System*™ please visit:

www.bodytype.com

Determine your bodytype online by selecting "Women's Test" or "Men's Test"

Give Your Senses The Joy Of
Spiritual Nutrition
With Chakra Harmony
Combine visual and sound toning techniques to harmonize your body, mind and spirit.

- Strengthen your energy field

- Balance your emotions

- Relieve stress

- Center yourself

- Feel more positive

- Clear your aura

- Transform suffering to joy

This easy to follow DVD shows you how to balance your life energies and relieve stress. Can be used actively or as a soothing background.

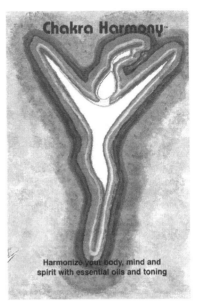

Harmonize your body, mind and spirit with essential oils and toning

---

Soft fabric travel pack kit with twelve 5/8 dram bottles containing 8 essential chakra oils:

Joy	Ylang Ylang
SARA	Cedarwood
Sacred Mountain	Release
White Angelica	Idaho Balsam Fir

Travel pack kit with 4 additional oils:

Frankincense	Peppermint
Peace & Calming	Purification

Chakra Harmony DVD	**$ 24.95**
Chakra Essential Oils Kit (8 Oils)	**119.95**
w/ Chakra Harmony DVD	**139.95**
Chakra Essential Oils Kit (12 Oils)	**159.95**
w/ Chakra Harmony DVD	**179.95**

Plus Shipping
Above items include quick reference card

Also Available
PEACEFUL WARRIOR TRAVEL PACK
$149.95
GUIDE TO PEACEFUL CONFLICT RESOLUTION
Peaceful Warrior Travel Pack contains 12 essential oils:

Peace & Calming	Purification	Peppermint	Frankincense
Valor	Lavender	Lemon	Harmony
Common Sense	Clarity	JuvaFlex	Highest Potential

Carolyn L. Mein, D.C.   P.O. Box 8112, Rancho Santa Fe, CA 92067
Phone: (858) 756-3704   Fax: (858) 756-6933
Visit *www.bodytype.com* for additional DVDs and resources

Made in the USA
San Bernardino, CA
16 November 2017